Children in Foster C

Researchers, practitioners, journalists and politicians increasingly complain that foster care throughout the world is in a state of crisis. There are more and more children needing care and, as residential alternatives dry up, more of these children are being assigned to foster families. This book reports the major findings of a two-year longitudinal study of 235 such children who entered the foster care system in South Australia between 1998 and 1999. As well as examining the changing policy context of children's services, the book documents the psychosocial outcomes for these children, their feedback on their experiences of care, and the views of their social workers and carers. In the process, the book examines some cherished beliefs about foster care policy and sheds new light on them.

The research reveals that, while most children do quite well in foster care up to the two-year point, there is a worrying amount of placement instability at a time when the concentration of emotionally troubled children in care is increasing throughout the western world. Although, surprisingly, placement instability does not appear to produce psychosocial impairment for a period of up to about one year in care, it has an extreme effect on children who are moved from placement to placement because no carer will tolerate their behaviour. These children are consigned to a life of disruption and emotional upheaval because of the lack of alternative forms of care. Another unexpected finding of the research is that increasing the rate of parental contact achieves little or nothing in relation to the likelihood of family reunification.

As child welfare increasingly enters a world of research-based practice, *Children in Foster Care* provides some much needed hard evidence of how foster care policy and practice can be improved.

James Barber is Dean of Social Work at the University of Toronto.
Paul Delfabbro is a Lecturer in Psychology at the University of Adelaide.

Children in Foster Care

James G. Barber
and Paul H. Delfabbro

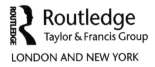

Routledge
Taylor & Francis Group

LONDON AND NEW YORK

First published 2004 by Routledge

2 Park Square, Milton Park, Abingdon, Oxfordshire OX14 4RN
52 Vanderbilt Avenue, New York, NY 10017

Routledge is an imprint of the Taylor & Francis Group, an informa business

First issued in paperback 2019

Typeset in 10/12pt Times New Roman
by Graphicraft Limited, Hong Kong

British Library Cataloguing in Publication Data
A catalogue record for this book is available
from the British Library

Library of Congress Cataloging in Publication Data
A catalog record for this book has been requested

ISBN 13: 978-0-415-31164-9 (hbk)
ISBN 13: 978-1-138-97035-9 (pbk)

Contents

Tables and figures

Tables

Figures

Foreword

Many organizations and fields are 'data-rich but information-poor' – a phrase used to describe the paucity of information that is concise and powerful enough to inform policy, administration and clinical services. In one respect, the field of foster care is both data-poor *and* information-poor. With the possible exception of Britain, most governments have not invested the resources necessary to address systematically the following basic questions:

- What forms of out-of-home care are most appropriate for specific types of children?
- What foster parent characteristics are associated with positive child development for what types of children?
- What factors predict foster home placement change or disruption?
- What strategies might be most effective for reunification for various sub-groups of families?
- What post-permanency supports are most crucial to provide?
- What are the long-term adult outcomes of various kinds of out-of-home care?
- What cultural and other diversity factors must be considered in programme design and implementation?
- What fiscal and legislative strategies encourage the most effective service delivery systems?
- What prevention strategies are most cost-effective for diverting families from the child welfare system?

In contrast, some organizations are so 'data-rich' that they are overloaded. These organizations, at least in parts of North America, are becoming overwhelmed with administrative data, the utility and limits of which are being recognized through the work of Chapin Hall, the University of California at Berkeley and the University of North Carolina at Chapel Hill, among others. Some states are concerned about the overwhelming amounts of data that these administrative information systems produce, their inability to effectively analyse and summarize what the data mean, and the continuing dearth of useful information about *specific interventions and indicators of child and family well-being.*

As a result of a lack of good information, practice myths are then confused with true practice wisdom, and intervention fads sweep the field. Instead, we should be concerned to develop careful practice approaches that stand the twin tests of their ability to be (1) cost-effectively replicated, and (2) reliably implemented with fidelity across workers and organizations in diverse communities.

Given this situation, we depend on independent evaluations such as the present study by James Barber and Paul Delfabbro to help fill crucial gaps in our knowledge base. These researchers have provided a valuable service by grounding their research in a cross-section of the foster care literature and practice policy from around the world to identify what is currently considered best practice.

What readers will find most valuable in this study is the way that the authors call into question some popular beliefs about effective practice, and how they maximize the utility of their study data to address key issues such as the effects of placement change, the relative importance of family contact, 'serial eviction' of children in care, and differing child perspectives about what affected them positively and negatively.

Experienced practitioners and researchers may find themselves challenged by what they read here. But this book will stimulate critical thinking about key practice issues, and encourage other studies that will directly test some of the practice myths that the authors are calling into question. The international review of major foster care literature, the use of standardized instruments, application of sophisticated data analysis approaches and cogent arguments about what the data mean are all reasons why expert evaluators and innovative administrators should read this book.

Peter J. Pecora

The Casey Family Programs, and
School of Social Work, University of Washington

Part I

An introduction to foster care

Chapter 1

Assessment, planning and intake

Introduction

In 1994 the world marked the International Year of the Family, and this fact alone is testament to the importance that cultures everywhere ascribe to the family. Like it or not, families are the most basic and enduring institution governing society. They mediate and interpret society to us as we grow to adulthood. More than this, family for most of us means home, and home, as Robert Frost once put it, 'is the place where, when you have to go there, they have to take you in' ('The Death of the Hired Hand'). But, for some children, the family home can be an impossible place to be. Sometimes the problem is abuse or neglect, sometimes it is parental illness, drug use or incapacity, and sometimes it is not a single problem but a combination of factors that means you'd better not go there, at least not at the moment. It is the mark of a civilized society that it provides alternative arrangements for children in this position, and it is the objective of such societies that they seek to make those arrangements as close as possible to the sanctuary that Robert Frost had in mind. In Australia, child protection is primarily the responsibility of state governments, and the child protection acts under which the states operate require the relevant Minister to ensure that all children have a satisfactory place to live. In theory, out-of-home care can take a variety of forms, and it can range in time from emergency care to long-term and even permanent care. In the main, however, out-of-home placements in Australia are primarily made with foster carers who are recruited, trained and supported by child welfare professionals.

One reason why family-based foster care deserves to be the preferred mode of temporary out-of-home care is because it is as close as you can get to the way most of us actually live. Besides, there is now considerable research evidence to suggest that conventional family-based care is the best option for most children (see, for example, McDonald *et al.* 1996; Minty 1999). Generally speaking, the research indicates that children from foster family care are more likely than children in group or institutional care to grow into well-functioning adults, as demonstrated by a wide range of social indicators such as high school completions, crime rates, drug and alcohol usage, divorce rates and satisfaction with life generally (Ferguson 1966; Festinger 1983; 1984). Festinger's (1983) study of 227 children who had been in foster care in New York, for example, found that most of those in long-term foster care during childhood became productive, law-abiding citizens in their early twenties. Similar findings have also been reported by Maluccio and Fein (1985), and by Zimmerman (1982). Of course correlational studies such as these prove nothing about the differential effectiveness of institutional versus foster family care as the two options normally cater for quite different populations. However, the fact that foster family care should generally be associated with positive outcomes (Fanshel and Shinn 1978) is cause for optimism, whatever may be said about the benefits of institutional care.

Australian foster carers are volunteer workers who are compensated for expenses incurred rather than paid an income. If a family-based foster placement cannot be provided, the child may be moved to a Community Residential Care (CRC) unit. These institutions are essentially diversionary programmes for young offenders and, if only for this reason, are normally seen as a last resort for children who are considered 'unfosterable'. As we shall see, however, CRCs regularly became home to foster children in our study. The least common form of alternative care is community-based housing, such as shared accommodation in subsidized housing, supervised placements with friends or neighbours, groups of siblings in subsidized housing, or mediated placements with extended family members.

Family-based foster care is not always an achievable option for children who must live apart from their parents. At various points in this book, we will refer to the distressing number of children in our study who had still not managed to find a stable foster home more than two years after being referred into care. The fundamental purpose of this book is to describe and learn from the experiences of these children as well as from the many success stories we witnessed in the course of the research. We begin our examination of foster care by reviewing the extant literature and practice policy from around the world in an effort to identify what is currently considered best practice in foster care. As we do this, it must be recognized that much of what is currently recommended is based on American research, and some authors have expressed scepticism about the portability of this work to other countries. Ainsworth (1997), for example, points out that the foster care population in the United States is dominated by children who are culturally dissimilar to Australian children in care. Moreover, there are significant legislative differences between Australia and the United States which have important implications for foster care practice. Generally speaking, child welfare policy throughout Australia places stricter limits on state intervention than exists in the USA. In most states of Australia, child protection legislation requires alternative care to be used as a short-term measure to ensure the safety of children or else to assist parents. As a consequence, adoption remains quite rare in Australia, with all states preferring to rely on temporary foster care in concert with interventions to reunify children with birth families. This is not to say that family reunification is required in all circumstances, of course. Child protection laws empower, indeed they compel, social workers to separate children from dangerous or negligent parents for as long as the situation remains perilous. But the existing policy preference in Australia is for separation to be temporary whenever possible and for every effort to be made to reunite children with their families of origin.

Notwithstanding this policy emphasis, the proclamation in late 2001 of the Children and Young Persons (Care and Protection) Amendment (Permanency Planning) Act in the state of New South Wales was a landmark in Australian foster care policy. In essence, these amendments represent a shift towards the American preference for 'permanency planning', which Fein, Maluccio, Hamilton and Ward (1983) have defined as 'a philosophy highlighting the value of rearing children in a family setting, preferably their biological families, [and] a theoretical framework stressing that stability and continuity of relationships promote children's growth and functioning' (p. 197). Permanency planning is intended to provide stability for every child who enters care, with a hierarchy of preferred options as follows: reunification with biological family, followed by adoption by foster carers or others, long-term foster care and residential placement as a last resort (Fein, Maluccio and Kluger 1990). Under the policy of permanency planning, social workers are to make time-limited plans at the point of intake for reunification *and* concurrent plans for adoption should family reunification prove impossible within a predetermined time period. In the United States, permanency planning received official sanction in the Adoption Assistance and Child Welfare Act (1980) which was a response to the alarming numbers of children who were experiencing harmful separations and indeterminate stays in care (cf. Barth and Berry 1987; Bryce and Ehlert 1971; Claburn, Magura and Resnick 1976; Katz 1990; Maluccio, Fein and Olmstead 1986). A further legislative attempt was made to keep children out of care in 1993 when the US Senate passed the Omnibus Budget Reconciliation Act (1993), which, *inter alia*, increased funding for family preservation services across the country. Further legislative support for the goal of permanency was provided by the Adoption and Safe Families Act (1997), the aim of which was to prevent children returning from foster care to unsafe homes and to find permanent homes for those unable to return to their biological families. Under this Act, a permanency planning hearing must be conducted within twelve months of placement for each child entering care and every twelve months thereafter (Gendell 2001). The state is required to petition for termination of parental rights in cases where a child has been in care for fifteen of the preceding twenty-two months (with some limited exceptions); where the court determines that a child has been abandoned; where parents have attempted to murder or have committed voluntary manslaughter of one of their children; or where parents have committed felony assault resulting in serious bodily harm to one of their children (Lindsey 2001). The Adoption and Safe Families Act also created financial incentives to state welfare departments to increase their rate of adoptions. A total of $US20 million was awarded each year until 2003 to states that led the nation in adoptions. Not surprisingly, children began moving out of the foster care system in large numbers. In the first year after the Act, for example, the numbers moving from foster care to adoption increased by almost 30 per cent, from 28,000 in 1996 to 36,000 in 1998 (Department of Health and Human Services 1999). It remains to be seen whether the permanency-planning amendments introduced recently in New South Wales will have a similar effect on the foster care population in that state but there is little doubt that the intention of the amendments is to move in this direction.

Notwithstanding international and, in Australia, *intra*national differences in foster care policy, there is general agreement around the world on the broad standards of care that should be provided to children in foster placement. In Australia, the Association of Children's Welfare Agencies' foster care standards extend to guidelines governing:

- thorough assessment prior to placement
- preparation for placement
- child–carer matching (including cultural background)
- written placement agreements between all the parties – carers, biological parents, the state and the child (according to age and capacity)
- contact with biological family
- carer training
- support worker case loads of no more than fifteen children, and
- placement follow-up and support.

(Association of Children's Welfare Agencies 1991)

Similarly, the Child Welfare League of America's 'blueprint' for fostering includes provisions for:

- strengths and needs assessment prior to placement
- supported transition to care
- involvement of children and families in case plans
- development of cultural and ethnic identity
- contact with biological family
- ongoing placement support, and
- carer and social worker training.

(Child Welfare League of America 1991)

In Britain, the National Foster Care Association's Charter (reproduced in Lowe 1991) states that high-quality foster care requires:

- a partnership model which includes the child where possible
- respect for cultural identity
- written agreements between the state and carers and biological parents, and
- carer and social worker training.

Principles and practice prescriptions such as these are ubiquitous in the literature, and while some, such as the need for comprehensive assessment, hardly require empirical justification, support for many entrenched practices can be difficult to find. In this chapter, we look at the literature relevant to foster care at the point before placement actually begins. We look first at the assessment of children and carers prior to placement before turning to practice recommendations regarding the behaviour of foster care support workers and the agencies that employ them. In this context, we consider the fundamental issues of co-ordination of support services and carer recruitment and training. Finally in this chapter, we look at some of the literature on preparation for placement. In the next chapter, we turn our attention to practice standards governing the placement itself.

Assessment principles

There is general agreement in the literature that not all children in need of out-of-home care are suitable for conventional family-based care. Outcome studies from the United States and Britain as well as data presented later in this book suggest that group home settings staffed by trained family care workers may well be a better option for children with severe behavioural or emotional disorders (see Chapter 10; Fratter *et al.* 1991; Hudson, Nutter and Galaway 1994; Whittaker, Tripodi and Grasso 1990). And in two recent Dutch studies, Scholte (1997) first compared the psychosocial characteristics of children in foster care with those in residential care, then in the second study he constructed a psychosocial profile of children who were forced to enter residential care because their foster placements had broken down. Both studies confirmed British and American experience that foster homes work best for younger children without clinically significant levels of emotional or behavioural disorder. Similarly, our own work (see Chapter 10) and that of many others (e.g. De Groot 1981; Fratter *et al.* 1991; Reeuwijk and Berben 1988; Stone and Stone 1983) shows that foster placements tend to be much more successful for young children than for emotionally troubled adolescents.

Thus, best practice in foster care should begin with a careful assessment of each child's suitability for placement. Where the child suffers from serious emotional or behavioural problems, regular foster care services are unlikely to be sufficient. Such children are likely to need either supervised group care or one of the forms of intensive, therapeutic foster care described in the literature (see Hudson, Natter and Galaway 1994, for a review). It is a cause for concern, therefore, that the trend in Australia generally has been towards a narrowing of placement options and an increasing reliance on conventional, family-based foster care (see Chapter 3).

Assessment of children

Assuming that foster care is a realistic option for the child, the next step in the assessment process needs to focus on the child's social, psychological and educational needs while in care. Among the most ambitious of the existing need assessment protocols is the Looking After Children (LAC) scheme developed by Parker *et al.* (1991) in Britain. LAC is one example of a movement across the United Kingdom, the United States, Canada and Australia towards standardized assessment and outcome-oriented case planning (American Humane Association 1993; Parker *et al.* 1991; Rapp and Poertner 1987). Briefly, LAC includes a series of 'Assessment and Action Records' designed for children in six age ranges in residential or foster care. Children are assessed on seven dimensions: health, education, identity, family and social relationships, social presentation, emotional and behavioural development, and self-care skills. Desired outcomes are specified for each dimension and questions are then asked about the actions needed to produce those outcomes. For example, it is known that children who are often read to in the early years are more likely to find reading easier, so one of the questions asked of carers of two- and three-year-old children concerns reading. If the answer is unsatisfactory, the caseworker is expected to take appropriate action. LAC also specifies a schedule for baseline and follow-up 'Action and Assessment' records.

Research and programme evaluation have been an integral part of the LAC project since its inception, and initial reports on its introduction in Britain, Canada, Sweden and Australia have been generally promising (Jones, Clark, Kufeldt and Norman 1998). Clare (1997), writing about the introduction of the Assessment and Action Records to Western Australia, for example, reported that LAC required only minor modifications to fit that state's legislation and practice. Further, practitioners and carers were generally positive about the system, particularly its potential to improve assessment, planning and review processes and accountability, and to enhance child-centred practice. Clare also noted the system's potential to provide a basis for practice standards, as well as data for planning and research.

In Victoria a pilot of LAC involving 37 children and young people was conducted by the Australian Institute of Family Studies (Wise 1999). Empirical evaluation was hampered by numerous threats to internal validity such as high staff turnover, competing demands on staff time, frequent placement changes and other events. Nevertheless, the author concluded that the materials required little adaptation, were generally accepted by those involved and were associated with modest improvements across a range of areas including the child's behaviour, education, relationships and physical health. On the other hand, Wise also identified impediments to the implementation of LAC in Australia including: an entrenched practice culture which emphasizes risk assessment at the expense of what happens in placement; the pressures of day-to-day practice and heavy case loads; and limited resources.

Thomas and O'Kane (1999) examined the extent to which children in care are involved in decision-making processes and found that use of LAC review forms was positively associated with children's participation in decision-making. Specifically, where LAC forms were used 63 per cent of children were invited to attend case planning meetings compared with 38 per cent in cases where the forms were not used. While it is sometimes said that the LAC review forms fail to qualify as outcome measures, their undoubted strength is that they compel social workers to perform a thoroughgoing intake assessment leading to a comprehensive case plan. So much so that Knight and Caveney (1998) have criticized LAC for being too painstaking, requiring practitioners to complete some thirty-five pages of questionnaire items for children under one year of age, and fifty-eight pages for young people over fifteen years of age. The authors also object that the instruments are shot through with class-based assumptions about what constitutes good parenting. Garrett (1999) goes further in his critique of the system, examining the socio-political context within which LAC was developed and adopted. He makes a number of observations, including: that LAC does not concern itself with the wider social issues confronted by many children and families; that 'looked after' children and 'reasonable parent' standards of care are not clearly defined; that LAC is based on an ideological view of young people and their world; and that the sample against which the LAC protocols were validated is unrepresentative of children in care. Garret also complained that the multiple-choice format of the Action and Assessment Records (375 questions for one age group) is directive and alienating and does not promote dialogue between social workers and clients. In fact, he sees the protocols as contributing to a bureaucratization of child protection social work (see also Knight and Caveney 1998), a situation which he warns deskills and deprofessionalizes child welfare work.

Similar concerns have been expressed by Bell (1998) as part of her report on the acceptability of LAC to those using the system. While she found that carers and young people in care were, for the most part, enthusiastic about the Action and Assessment Records, she found social workers were in two minds about their usefulness. On the one hand, the Records were seen as having the potential to enhance professional decisions but, on the other hand, it was felt that they had the potential to impose artificial boundaries on potential interventions.

Notwithstanding such criticisms of Looking After Children, structured need assessment protocols deserve to be part of any best practice approach to foster care because they promote consistency and comprehensiveness in case planning.

Assessment of carers

Another commonly advocated aspect of assessment concerns the match between potential carer and foster child. Intuitively, this seems an uncontentious proposition but, after reviewing the literature on factors associated with placement breakdown, Teather, Davidson and Pecora (1999) noted that comparatively little research has been conducted in this area and they caution that individual difference factors probably do not make a critical difference. Rather, they suggest, it is the complex interplay between carer, child and social worker characteristics, and, quite probably, broader societal and institutional factors as well, that determine placement success.

Orme and Buehler (2001) conducted an exhaustive review of the literature on foster family characteristics, and one of their major findings was that very few studies shed any light on which foster environments are most beneficial to children in care. Indeed, their search of all papers published in this area since 1965 yielded a total of only thirty-four studies. Most were cross-sectional, involved small and/or unrepresentative samples, did not employ random assignment and lacked control or even comparison groups. Not only is the process of carer–child matching made more difficult by the paucity of research findings, but it is further hampered by the fact that most of the research that has been undertaken has involved female carers only, even when they are part of a two-parent household.

Nevertheless, some guidelines for placement selection can be extracted from the literature with a reasonable degree of confidence. For example Dando and Minty (1987) interviewed 80 foster carers to determine their motives for caring, their backgrounds and their attitudes to fostering. Social workers rated the carers across various dimensions to arrive at three categories: very good performance, good performance and reservations about performance. Two sub-groups emerged among those rated as successful foster carers: childless couples and female carers who, from personal experience, identified with deprived or damaged children. Women who were motivated by altruism or social conscience also rated well whereas women whose motivation was that they 'like children' were not highly rated.

It has also been established that several carer traits are associated with poor outcomes. Among them are authoritarian child-rearing styles, possessiveness towards the foster child, more highly educated carers (Sanchirico et al. 1998) and the belief that child development is entirely dependent on heredity (Wit and Adriani 1971; Van der Oever, Hoogheid and Hirschfeldt 1979). Rowe (1976) found that foster carers who are more tolerant of a child's difficult behaviour or poor academic performance are more successful than less tolerant foster carers. His findings also suggested that social class was not related to quality of care and that a low demand on children for religious observance was associated with successful placement.

Sandow (1998) examined 42 carer–child relationships and found that parenting skills, empathy on the part of the carer and the carer's ability to recognize and deal with the child's losses were associated with positive relationships and improvement by the child while in placement. Several child-related variables, notably a higher level of social competence and fewer behavioural problems, were also associated with better carer–child relationships. A small study of 14 specialist foster carers (Ray and Horner 1990) found that the more successful female carers were likely to be enthusiastic, to demonstrate maturity, to be able to face reality and to make decisions based on logic.

Cautley and Aldridge (1975) interviewed 963 applicants for foster children, and 115 of the families approved as carers were interviewed periodically to identify determinants of successful foster parenting. Social workers' ratings of the placement and of the female carer (the male carers were not well enough known by the social workers to be rated) were used as indicators of placement success. It was found that it is preferable for the foster child to be the youngest child in the home and that a pre-school child or children in the home is a negative factor. Further, for female carers, being the eldest child was associated with success while, for male carers, being the eldest or only child was negatively associated with success. In general, higher levels of parenting skills, understanding, coping with difficult behaviour, co-operation with the social worker, flexibility and concern for the foster child were also shown to be predictive of successful placement.

Common sense would suggest that the temperamental match between carer and child is at least as important as other carer characteristics but, again, it is difficult to extract practice guidelines from the limited research conducted in this area. For example, Green, Braley and Kisor (1996) found that when temperamentally 'easy' children were matched with carers of similar temperament, the carers reported higher family functioning and better foster care adjustment than in unmatched cases. Not surprisingly, the optimal combinations were found to be flexible female carers and 'positive-mood' adolescents, and positive-mood male carers and positive-mood adolescents. Complicating this picture, however, was the fact that, if adolescents' and case managers' reports of family functioning and adjustment were used instead of carers' reports, these findings were not supported. In a study by Doelling and Johnson (1990) correlation analyses showed particularly poor outcomes for the combination of negative mood in the child and authoritarianism in the female carer.

It would also seem sensible to accommodate carer preferences in respect of age, sex and background of child they would like to foster. In their survey of United States and Canadian agencies providing Therapeutic Foster Care, Snodgrass and Bryant (1989) found that 74 per cent of agencies consider

carer preferences when placing children. Agencies may also consider matching a carer's experience and expertise with the child's needs, as well as
matching according to culture, proximity to biological family and the child's
preference for rural or urban setting. Equally, it is important to accommodate foster child preferences wherever possible, and studies which have reported the views of children and young people in care lend firm support to
this proposition (Community Services Commission 2000b; Festinger 1983;
Johnson, Yoken and Voss 1995).

Co-ordination of support services

There is clearly no point conducting an entry-to-care assessment if it is not
connected to a service delivery system. Moreover, an ever-increasing number
of children entering the alternative care system have multiple needs span-
ning more than one agency's jurisdiction (see also Chapter 10). It is not
uncommon, for example, for foster children to have been abused at home,
to have committed a crime themselves, to be unruly at school *and* to suffer
a severe emotional or behavioural disorder of some kind. It is essential
therefore that multi-problem children obtain access to services across multiple systems. Despite this, American research suggests that, although foster
children are among the unhealthiest in that country, they utilize the health
system less than children from the general population (Aday and Anderson
1975; Combs-Orme, Chernoff and Kager 1991; Klee and Halfon 1987).

In recognition of this problem, the state of Tennessee in the United States
created six-person service co-ordination teams to assume responsibility for
children entering state custody. Irrespective of how the children entered
state care, whether through mental health services, juvenile justice, child
protection or educational services, for example, the teams were given the
authority to obtain services and placements from any agency. The service
co-ordination teams were independent of the service delivery systems and
were responsible for the assessment, residential placement, referral to appropriate services and monitoring of the child's progress while in the care
of the state. The service co-ordination teams selected which agency should
assume primary responsibility for the case and which agencies should be
required to provide additional support services. In a quasi-experimental
evaluation of this system, Glisson (1994) randomly selected 300 children
entering state custody from counties where the service teams were trialled,
and compared them with 300 randomly selected children entering custody
from non-participating counties. Among Glisson's findings were that service
co-ordination teams improved access to mental health services for clinically
disturbed children, and, perhaps as a result, the most seriously disturbed
children showed greater improvement in service co-ordination counties. In
addition, service co-ordination teams used significantly fewer restrictive placement options for the children in their care.

More than a decade ago, the Child Welfare League of America (CWLA) (1988) promulgated a set of health care standards for children in out-of-home care. Among the recommendations contained in those standards were entry-point health assessments for all children entering foster care, consisting of comprehensive health, mental health and developmental assessments within thirty days of placement into care. The standards also insist on guaranteed access to ongoing health care in placement, agency administration mechanisms, including centralized health services management units with responsibility for the health of children in care, and the creation of a centralized health information database covering all children in care. The standards also mandate basic first-aid training for foster parents and caseworkers. Finally, the standards emphasize the need for adequate co-ordination of services, including but not restricted to health care services for every child.

Less than a year after the CWLA set out its standards, the state of California launched a comprehensive programme of service delivery and legislative change to give effect to the recommendations (Klee, Soman and Halfon 1992). Among the programme initiatives was a Foster Youth Services programme which worked through schools to track down foster children's student records to verify that their immunizations were current. The same programme provided academic tutoring and offered counselling and consultation regarding the children's academic performance. A Partners-in-Care Program sponsored quarterly education training seminars for carers of medically fragile children. A court-appointed Special Advocate programme mobilized volunteers to monitor the progress of children under court orders and provide findings and recommendations directly to the court. Among the state's legislative initiatives was the California Senate Bill 370 which required the development of a mental health needs assessment protocol for children in care. The California Assembly Bill 2268 established foster homes for children with special health needs, including specialized care payment rates and training for foster parents.

While the Californian programme appears most impressive, a similar case planning system known as the Fostering Individualized Assistance Program (FIAP) was evaluated by Clark et al. (1993) and found to be little more effective than conventional family-based care. Like the Californian system, FIAP was an individualized, case-managed and collaborative intervention for children in the welfare system. It involved strengths-based assessment, life-domain planning, clinical case-management and supports and services. One hundred and seven children aged seven to fifteen, in care for child protection reasons, were randomly assigned to FIAP or standard practice conditions. There were no significant differences between the two groups on measures of the children's behaviour at baseline. Both groups improved significantly over eighteen months, with the treatment group showing more improvement in emotional and behavioural adjustment than the standard practice group.

If the ultimate objective of foster placement is to reunite children with their parents, then comprehensive service planning must extend beyond the child to include his or her family of origin as well. Lawder, Poulin and Andrews (1986), for example, found that a significant amount of the variance in reunification rates was accounted for by parent-of-origin variables, particularly teenage parenthood and the existence of mental health problems. And Gambrill and Wiltse (1974) discovered that early return home is associated with goal-oriented worker–parent contacts, and working agreements between worker and parent. It follows that no amount of intervention with the child is likely to be effective in facilitating reunification unless the family-of-origin environment is assessed and modified as necessary.

Social worker and agency characteristics

Some studies have suggested that the child's social worker plays a vital role in the success or otherwise of foster care (Cautley and Aldridge 1975; Hess, Folaron and Jefferson 1992). One crucial consideration seems to be the rate of contact between social workers and families of origin. For example, Boyd's (1979) eighteen-month pilot project trained volunteers who took over routine jobs such as clerical work and client transportation so that social workers could increase the amount of time they spent with families of origin. Results of this quasi-experiment showed a dramatic decrease in social worker case loads because of the increased number of foster children who were returned home during that time.

In a study of the stability of 64 placements, Stone and Stone (1983) gathered data on caseworker, child, natural parent and foster carer characteristics, as well as information on agency–family contacts. It was found that caseworker input (degree of contact, rapport building and energy expended on the case) was the variable most strongly associated with placement success. Sanchirico et al.'s (1998) survey of 616 carers also found a positive correlation between in-person contact with caseworker and carer job satisfaction. More important to job satisfaction, yet associated with caseworker involvement, was the quality of the carer's involvement in service planning. Shapiro (1976) found that high frequency of caseworker contact, experience, stability and low case loads strongly influenced discharge rate during the first two years of placement, but the influence of these factors declined from that point.

Bilson and Barker's (1995) British study of children in care found that social work contact decreased rapidly after the first six months in care, infrequent contact being associated with stable placement (see also Chapter 11). The authors warn that, apart from the need for social workers to monitor the placement, apparently stable placements may break down when the child reaches adolescence and the social worker is disadvantaged by the lack of an ongoing relationship.

Carer recruitment and training

For decades now, complaints have regularly appeared in the literature about the shortage of suitable foster carers throughout the western world (Govan 1951; Taylor and Starr 1967; Carbino 1980; Lawrence 1994). One reason for the low success of recruitment campaigns is suggested by an Australian study in which 91 people who enquired about fostering children were followed up by telephone survey (Keogh and Svensson 1999). It was found that, of the 96 per cent who had decided against fostering, half made the decision for personal reasons, but half reported that they had been discouraged by the response they received when contacting the agency.

Smith and Gutheil (1988) reported on a recruitment programme run by the Salvation Army in New York City. At the end of the first year, the programme had increased the number of placements by 49 per cent, compared with 6 per cent for New York City overall. It was found that personal recruitment by friends or family already fostering was more effective than recruiting via the media, and trained recruiters were more successful than untrained recruiters.

A US survey of prospective foster carers attending a twelve-hour fostering preparation course examined influences on the decision to foster or not to foster (Baum, Crase and Crase 2001). Of the respondents, 315 (64 per cent of the total attending) completed the survey prior to training and 182 (58 per cent of the 313) completed the survey six months after the training. Survey questions asked what aspects of the training method and course content had influenced the decision to foster or not to foster, and what factors other than training had influenced the decision. The range of responses was broad and, while training content was reported to be useful, fewer than 10 per cent of respondents said that it influenced their decision to foster. More important influences included responding to the need for more carers (31 per cent), the fostering experience of family or friends (21 per cent) and the wish to expand the family (19 per cent).

A comprehensive study of carer recruitment and retention was conducted by the Casey Family Program (Casey Family Program 2000), which concluded that there are ten pre-placement practice principles that should guide foster care practice:

1 Develop clear agency values, assumptions and goals
2 Create organizational structures that facilitate good practice
3 Seek and build collaborations
4 Clarify roles and responsibilities
5 Emphasize responsiveness and inclusivity in recruitment (i.e. be prepared to adjust licensing requirements in the interests of finding the best placement for each child)
6 Help families to be competent

7 Find the right family for the right child (multi-faceted matching)
8 Support teamwork and partnerships between social workers, carers and birth families
9 Provide sufficient concrete and emotional support to carers
10 Give families a voice in the system.

According to the Case Family Program, such principles should maximize the number of carers recruited and minimize carer attrition.

A common feature of foster carer training programmes is a lack of evaluation of their effectiveness (Berry 1988), but most of the available evidence suggests that foster carers are hungry for pre- and in-service training. Gilligan (1996) mailed thirty-six-item questionnaires to all foster carers in one largely rural health board region in Ireland and received completed questionnaires from 73 respondents (54.4 per cent). Twenty-nine per cent of respondents reported difficulty in managing disruptive behaviour and 43 per cent did not know how to respond to a child talking about painful past experiences. Almost half of the respondents said that they did not understand the child in their care. And in Wells and D'Angelo's (1994) study of 40 specialized foster carers, training was one of the specific areas in which respondents requested agency support.

In response to carer demand, the National Foster Care Association (NFCA) in Britain developed an introductory course for foster carers it released under the title *The Challenge of Foster Care* (Berkley-Hill 1988) and it soon became the standard for foster care training throughout the UK. The training programme centres on the NFCA's Foster Care Charter, the key underpinnings of which include respect for biological parents, equal status of carers and agency workers, and commitment to task-centred foster care. According to Lowe (1991: 153):

> The training program encourages prospective and existing carers to see themselves as an integral part of the child care team. Clear placement goals, access to information, adequate support, continuing training opportunities, an active role in decision-making, and adequate financial rewards are theirs [the carers'] as a right.

While the need for training and support is frequently identified, outcomes of training programmes are less frequently documented. Among the programmes that have been evaluated is one providing training to carers of infants suffering prenatal drug effects and whose care therefore requires specialized knowledge and skills (Burry 1999). Subjects self-selected for specialized training or regionally televised training. Those in the specialized training group demonstrated superior knowledge of the effects of substances on infants and enhanced skills in handling these babies. There was, however, no change in either group's feelings of efficacy or intent to foster a substance-affected child.

Boyd and Remy (1978) examined 267 placements involving 120 foster families in which one or both parents were trained. Training was a behaviourally oriented sixteen-week programme complemented (for families with the highest-risk children) by in-home visits. Placements were categorized according to duration (up to or longer than two years) and whether carers were trained or untrained. Trained foster carers tended to be more experienced (i.e. licensed longer) than untrained carers although they did not have a higher proportion of high-risk children. Foster child characteristics prompted carers to undergo training. Using multiple regression analysis, it was found that training had a weak but significant effect on placement outcomes independent of foster carer experience, placement stress or child characteristics. From these results it was estimated that training would result in a higher number of carers retaining their licences.

Barth, Yeaton and Winterfelt (1994) evaluated an eleven-session support, education and training programme for carers of sexually abused children. There were two treatment groups: one for relative carers and the other for non-relative carers; the total in both groups was 15 carers. The control group comprised 12 carers of sexually abused children. The carers who attended the sessions unanimously reported that they had learned ways to care for and manage their foster child but there was no improvement in the children's sexualized behaviour.

A randomized controlled trial in 17 local council areas in Scotland evaluated the impact of carer training on children's emotional and behavioural functioning (Minnis et al. 2001). A total of 121 carers of 182 children were randomly allocated to either standard services or standard services plus additional training. The training course comprised three six-hour sessions over one week. Pre- and post-training measures of child psychopathology and functioning were obtained, and carers in the training condition evaluated the programme. They reported that they derived substantial benefit from the programme and that the child in their care was better behaved. However, on formal measures there was no change in the level of child psychopathology.

Meadowcroft and Grealish (1990) suggest that one measure of the success of carer training and support should be the length of time carers remain in service. However, in their report on retention of treatment parents in the PRYDE Therapeutic Foster Care programme which provides intensive pre-service and in-service training, they note that, even with intensive training, specialist carers do not remain in service for as long as non-professional carers do.

Preparation for placement

Foster carers around the western world repeatedly call for better preparation prior to placement. Wells and D'Angelo (1994), for example, conducted focus groups with forty specialized foster carers who identified placement preparation as crucial to their understanding of a child's behaviour and, consequently, to the care they provide. They also called for preparation for placement termination, as abrupt transitions can be distressing to carer and child alike.

Smith (1994) circulated a brief questionnaire to carers who had experienced placement disruption and received 31 responses covering 38 children. Respondents' perceptions of the cause of placement breakdown were: lack of information, inadequate assessment of the child and behaviour problems. Carers frequently reported that they had difficulty in understanding and dealing with the child's behaviour. And when asked about preparation for placement some families said that, had they understood the extent of the demands on them, they might not have proceeded. Almost all respondents felt guilt and failure after placement disruption.

In a retrospective multiple regression study of 184 children, Palmer (1996) found that including parents in the transition to foster care was significantly associated with placement stability. More specifically, Palmer found that, if the parent was actively involved in preparing the child for the move, the placement was less likely to break down. Cautley and Aldridge (1975) found that preparation of the foster parents by the social worker prior to placement is important to placement success, that several contacts are preferable and that at least one contact should include the male carer.

In a retrospective study of birth parents, foster carers, children in care and social workers (Kufeldt, Armstrong and Dorosh 1996), it was found that birth parents did not usually accompany their child to placement, even when placement was with parental agreement. From their knowledge of practice in other countries, the authors suggested that whether or not parents accompany children to placement depends on whether inclusive or exclusive models of fostering are followed. Of course, it is necessary to differentiate between placements for which there is parental agreement and those which occur against parents' wishes as part of child protection proceedings. In Australia, 91 per cent of children in out-of-home care are under a court order (Australian Institute of Health and Welfare 2000) and a number of these orders are contested by the parents. When children are placed without parental co-operation, then, ensuring the safety of children and carers may preclude placement preview or parental contact with foster carers.

Studies suggest that foster children themselves normally want some form of preparation for placement. Johnson, Yoken and Voss (1995) interviewed fifty-nine children in care and found that they thought carers should know before placement about the child's history and reasons for placement, as well as the child's personality, likes and dislikes, etc. Trial visits to prospective foster homes before deciding whether to proceed with the placement were among the suggestions made by young people who had been in care (Festinger 1983). A consultation with Australian children and young people in care (Community Services Commission 2000) produced the recommendation that children's personal and placement preferences should be taken into account when potential carers are considered, and that several carer–child contacts should take place before a final placement decision is made. Acknowledging the distress and confusion children and young people may experience in the case of an emergency placement, alternative care procedures in New South Wales make several provisions aimed at mitigating the distress. Among them are that the child should be accompanied to placement by their social worker or someone they know, and this person should stay with the child for some time during the transition period. The child should also be provided with full information about the reason for and expected duration of the placement (New South Wales Department of Community Services 1998).

While there is little compelling evidence that placement preparation influences placement outcomes, it nevertheless seems reasonable to assume that the child's emotional well-being, at least in the short term, is best served by some form of preparation. A gradual planned introduction to the carer and the new home has the potential to ease the anxiety inevitably experienced by a child in what is often an unwelcome transition to an unfamiliar environment.

Summary

In summary, a feature of the existing literature on foster care assessment, intake and planning is that much of it is descriptive rather than evaluative. Research studies typically involve small, unrepresentative samples, and many are correlational in nature. Notwithstanding limitations in the available data, a number of practice guidelines can be extracted from the extant literature with at least some degree of confidence. Propositions for which there is a moderate degree of empirical support include the following:

- Some children are unsuitable for conventional family-based foster care and should be screened out. Adolescents with conduct and/or mental health problems are particularly poorly suited and require more intensive or residential options (see also Chapter 11).
- Comprehensive baseline assessments using structured protocols promote comprehensive case planning.
- All things being equal, it is better for the foster child to be the youngest in the house.
- Service co-ordination teams improve foster child access to services.
- Personal contact by current carers is among the more effective methods of recruiting new carers.
- Pre-service training is subjectively important to carers.
- Placement outcomes are normally better when the biological parent is involved in the transition to care.

- Providing pre-placement information to the child eases the anxiety associated with the move.
- Young people themselves want pre-placement preparation and involvement in the placement decision.

Among characteristics of foster carers that have been associated with successful placements are:

- non-authoritarian child-rearing styles
- non-possessiveness towards the foster child
- rejection of the belief that child development is dependent on heredity
- tolerance of difficult behaviour and poor academic performance
- low demand on children for religious observance
- female carers who, from personal experience, identify with deprived or damaged children.

Social worker or agency characteristics associated with good placement outcomes and carer satisfaction include:

- regular contact with the carer
- providing the carer with adequate pre-placement information
- keeping the carer informed and involved in case planning.

Propositions for which the evidence is weak or mixed but which are commonly put forward in the literature on foster care include the following:

- There is an optimal match in carer–child characteristics.
- Foster carer pre-training improves placement retention or placement outcomes.

In the next chapter, we examine practice standards relating to the next stage of foster care – the stage after the child actually arrives in care.

Chapter 2

In-care standards

Introduction

The previous chapter showed that, by the time a child arrives in care, a great deal of thought and work should already have been done. In this chapter we turn to the attributes of the placement itself that are commonly said to be associated with successful outcomes. As with the previous chapter we will find that there is a high degree of consensus in the field which is not altogether justified by the strength of the available evidence. We begin by considering interventions for the promotion of stable foster placements before turning to the potential role of the biological family in foster care through sibling co-placement, kinship care and parental visiting. We then consider methods for dealing with separation distress, foster carer support and remuneration and external case review before finishing with a brief overview of the issues involved in planning for discharge.

Placement stability

This issue of placement stability is the subject of a later chapter, so the empirical arguments for and against permanency planning can be deferred until then. At this stage, we can confine our attention to foster care programmes intended to minimize placement disruption. One such programme that targets twelve- to eighteen-year-olds with a history of placement disruption and problem behaviour has been described and evaluated by Taber and Proch (1987). In this study, the authors tracked the placement stability of 51 young people accepted into the programme, and for each case they assembled a planning team consisting of the young person, significant others, the assessing clinician, a social worker and a programme staff member. After placement, the team expanded to include the agency social worker and the young person's care givers. Foster children were actively involved in case planning and attended all meetings at which their case was discussed. A comprehensive assessment identified the young person's developmental needs and the services required for a stable placement, and a 'service prescription' formed the basis of placement negotiation. The situation was carefully monitored after placement and the care giver was offered support and access to consultation. Taber and Proch's (1987) evaluation showed that young people in the programme had an average of 1.8 moves after the programme compared with 4.8 prior to intervention. Furthermore, prior to intervention 70 per cent of placements had been in institutions; after the intervention this figure fell to 19 per cent.

Katz (1990) has described another promising approach to promoting placement stability among severely dysfunctional families. This programme applies five major permanency planning methods from existing child welfare knowledge. Firstly, social workers have reduced case loads (a maximum of ten). Secondly, there is early case planning, under which principle every case should have clearly written goals and timelines (see pp. 3–7). Thirdly, because parents' own problems are the reason for placement, intensive services to parents are provided by weekly in-person casework. Fourthly, short-term written contracts are drawn up with parents to make clear precisely what is being asked of them before their children can be returned. Finally, the contract also specifies weekly visits between biological parents and their children. The results of Katz's project were that most of the children achieved permanency but almost none of them with biological parents. Nevertheless, Katz claimed success for the programme because it achieved permanency for children from extremely disturbed families who had previously experienced frequent disruption and placement change.

Sibling co-placement

There is general consensus in the literature that it is normally better to place siblings together rather than separate them (e.g. Kosonen 1996). Despite this, Staff and Fein's (1992) comparison of placement breakdown rates for siblings placed together versus separately did not find any advantage in sibling co-placement overall, and, in the case of white children, placement breakdown was actually higher under conditions of co-placement. In contrast, Thorpe and Swart (1992) and Berridge and Cleaver (1987) have reported lower breakdown rates under conditions of co-placement, and Grigsby (1994) has reported shorter placement duration for children placed with siblings.

Part of the problem with the research evidence results from confusion about how to count placement breakdown in the case of siblings. For example, when siblings are placed together and the placement breaks down, should that count as one breakdown or two? Staff and Fein's (1992) work suggests that, when the measure is defined as the number of individual children disrupted, co-placement does not necessarily produce better outcomes. A further problem with the research evidence is that, because children are never randomly assigned to placement conditions, it is impossible to be definitive about the preferable placement type.

Placement breakdown is only one measure of failure, of course, and studies which have explored the experiences of children who have been in care (Millham *et al.* 1986; Farmer and Parker 1991; Bullock, Little and Millham 1993; Community Services Commission 2000) invariably report that most children in foster care value their sibling relationships very highly and long to maintain them. Hegar (1988) reviewed the literature on sibling loss and separation and recommended co-placement of children in care wherever possible. Her recommendation was influenced by research suggesting that close sibling access and relationships are important both in childhood and in adulthood. Similarly, studies exploring the experiences of adults who grew up in foster or institutional care consistently record the sadness of respondents when they recall their experiences of separation from brothers and sisters (Ferguson 1966; Meier 1966; Triseliotis 1980; Triseliotis and Russell 1984). Unless there are very good reasons to the contrary, then, every effort should be made to place siblings together.

Extended family (kinship) care

It is standard practice in foster care services throughout the western world to prefer out-of-home placements with relatives to non-relative foster care. In the United States, the number of children in 'kinship foster care' has been rising rapidly over the last decade or so. In a survey of 25 states back in 1992, Kusserow (1992) reported that the percentage of children in kinship care had grown from 18 per cent in 1986 to 31 per cent in 1990. And in Illinois and New York City, around half of all children in care were in 1994 in the care of relatives (Dubowitz 1994). Because of differences in the way the data are collected, it is difficult to compare Australian and American figures directly, but in Australia around a third of all foster children are recorded as being in extended family care (Australian Institute of Health and Welfare 2000). This figure varies between states and territories, with New South Wales having the highest proportion at 51 per cent and South Australia the lowest at 10 per cent (Australian Institute of Health and Welfare 2000).

Despite the current preference for extended family care, there is little evidence in support of the practice, and findings from the studies that have been conducted are actually quite mixed. The positive features of care by relatives often include the availability of additional placement resources, a setting with which the child is likely to be familiar and carers whose commitment to the child may be stronger than that of strangers. When placement is with relatives, there is the added likelihood that children may feel the pain of separation from biological parents less acutely. The evidence for these beliefs is for the most part indirect and anecdotal rather than systematic (Berrick and Barth 1994), although recent research suggests a greater sense of security for children placed with relatives than for those placed with non-relatives. And in a study of 1,100 children in out-of-home care, Wilson and Conroy (1999) found that 94 per cent of those in care with relatives reported always feeling loved compared with 82 per cent of those in care with non-relatives.

On the other hand, concern has been raised about the quality of extended family homes since they, after all, are the very families that helped to produce the child's troubled parents in the first place (Dubowitz, Feigelman and Zuravin 1993; General Accounting Office 1995). Furthermore, the physical environment may be of a lower standard than non-family placements (Berrick 1997), and relative carers have been found to experience depression (Fuller-Thomson and Minkler 2000) and other psychological problems (Robinson, Kropf and Myers 2000) more often than non-relative carers. Fein and Maluccio (1984) also note that placement with relatives can be abused in order to save funds, and can overburden relatives with children who have special needs.

Courtney (1996) reported on all children who entered foster care in California in 1988, and whose progress was followed up to 1992. He found that kinship care proved to be a comparatively stable environment in that children moved around less often than those in unrelated foster family homes. Among 'closed cases', for example, children placed in foster family homes averaged 2.01 placements over the four years, compared with 1.45 placements for children placed with relatives. Among open cases, children who were first placed in foster homes averaged 2.98 placements, compared with those placed with kin, who had 1.85 placements. And among those cases that remained open for the entire three-to-four-year study period, about 63 per cent of children placed initially with relatives remained with the same caretaker, and 80 per cent had no more than two caretakers. In contrast, among children initially placed in foster homes, almost 79 per cent of open cases had experienced at least two and 49 per cent at least three placements by the end of four years. Part of the explanation for this last finding is that a larger proportion of children in extended family care were permanently placed with them. Numerous other studies confirm that kinship placements last longer and that reunification rates are lower than traditional foster placements (e.g. Berrick, Barth and Needle 1994; Everett 1995; Scannapieco, Hegar and McAlpine 1997; Tam and Ho 1996; Usher, Randolph and Gogan 1999; Wulczyn and Goerge 1992).

Courtney and Barth (1996) found that final placement with relatives was associated with successful exit from foster care, but little is known about longer-term outcomes for children in kinship care (see also Link 1996). In one United States study, however, Benedict, Zuravin and Stallings (1996) interviewed 214 young adults who had spent time in foster care, 86 of whom had spent most of their time in foster care with relatives and 128 of whom had been in non-relative foster care. Results indicated that there were no significant differences between the two groups on measures of education, employment, income, housing stability, history of homelessness, stress or social support. There was, however, a difference between the groups on heroin use, with 28 per cent of the relative care group and 11 per cent of the non-relative group reporting that they had used the drug at some time.

In their study of kinship care in one Maryland county, Scannapieco, Hegar and McAlpine (1997) compared all 33 kinship placements with a 40 per cent random sample of the population of 140 traditional foster placements. The authors found that children in traditional foster care received significantly more mental health and transportation services than children in kinship care. On the other hand, children in kinship care received significantly more substance-abuse treatment. It is impossible to know whether these differences reflect discrepancies between relative and non-relative carers in respect of family circumstances or access to services, or whether they reflect differences in the populations of children. However, the available evidence suggests that children in kinship care do receive less assistance from child welfare authorities (Dubowitz, Feigelman and Zuravin 1993). Moreover, recent qualitative research by Davidson (1997) involving thirty kinship carers suggests that they felt deprived of basic household items such as beds, food, personal hygiene items and toys as well as access to support services such as respite care and transport. In view of these findings, it seems prudent to suggest that, if kinship care is to be the preferred option, steps should be taken to ensure that carers are guaranteed access to all of the services available to traditional foster carers.

Large differences between relative and non-relative placements in relation to parent–child contact have been reported by Le Prohn (1994), who compared the role perceptions of relative and non-relative foster carers. Eighty-two relative care families and 98 non-relative care families with the United States' Casey Family Program were included in the study. Relative carers identified more strongly than non-relative carers with the parenting role and as facilitators of the child's contact with birth family. Using data from the same study, Le Prohn and Pecora (1994) found that children in relative placements had much more contact with biological family. Of children whose parents' whereabouts were known, the mean number of contacts with their mother was 35 a year, compared with 4 contacts for children in non-relative placements. Similarly, the mean number of child–father contacts for children in relative care was 16, compared with 2 for children in non-relative care. There was also a marked difference in sibling contact. The numbers of children in relative and non-relative care who ever saw siblings were the same, but those living with relatives had an average of 90 visits a year compared with 14 visits a year for those in other placements. In the absence of random assignment, however, it is impossible to know whether this effect is attributable to relative care or selection bias.

Parental visiting

Among the most reliably reported findings in the foster care literature is the connection between, on the one hand, the frequency and reliability of parental visiting and, on the other, shorter time in foster care or family reunification (Gibson, Tracy and DeBord 1984; Lawder, Poulin and Andrews 1986; Mech 1985; see also Chapter 8). In his five-year longitudinal study, for example, Fanshel (1975) showed that parental visiting was the single best predictor of foster children returning to their original homes. Conversely, discussing her studies of children in care, Swedish researcher Andersson (1999) postulates that for some children parental visiting may be the key to successful foster placement in that it demonstrates the parents' acceptance of the fostering arrangement and shows the child that 'both sides accept each other' (p. 183).

A significant association has been found between parental visiting and a number of measures of child well-being (Cantos, Gries and Slis 1997; Fanshell and Shinn 1978; Poulin 1985). Poulin (1992), for example, studied 92 children in long-term care to examine the relationship between family visiting and the child's attachment to biological family. It was found that family attachment and identification are higher when biological family remain involved in the child's life, although the author noted that the sample was drawn from one agency and may not be representative of the population of young people in care. Despite the correlational nature of this research, such findings have led many practitioners to press strongly for parental visits as an indispensable component of care planning (e.g. Hess 1982; Hess et al. 1992). On a cautionary note, however, the American Academy of Pediatrics' Committee on Early Childhood recently noted that problems often attend parental visits and that not just any kind of contact will do (Miller et al. 2000). As the risks and benefits of parental visiting are the subject of another chapter (see Chapter 8), we can defer further discussion of this issue until then. At this stage, however, it is important to note that one compelling reason for promoting parental visiting is that the majority of children in foster care want it (Rest and Watson 1984; Kufeldt 1984). For example, Johnson, Yoken and Voss (1995) interviewed 59 children aged from eleven to fourteen years who had been in family foster care for between six and twenty-four months at the time of interview. While 73 per cent reported that they got along well with their foster carers, all but three respondents said they missed their families and 56 per cent reported missing their parents most of the time. An Australian survey of 66 children in care (Community Services Commission 2000) found that 47 respondents wanted more contact with family and other significant people, and all but 5 nominated someone whom they no longer saw but would have liked to. A British study which elicited the views of 45 young people on various aspects of foster care found that their wishes on parental contact were usually not heeded (Buchanan

1995). In a retrospective study involving 92 children in foster care, their mothers, female foster carers and social workers (Kufeldt, Armstrong and Dorosh 1996), it was found that 89 per cent of children and 79 per cent of parents believed that the child's going into care had been the best solution. Even though foster and birth families were reportedly in favour of contacting each other and working together, 33 per cent of children and 40 per cent of parents wanted more visits.

One approach to promoting parental visiting has been described by Simms and Bolden (1991). In this Family Reunification Program, biological parents are provided with transport to a neutral setting – a Child Guidance Clinic – in which a structured visit takes place with their child. The first hour of the visit consists of a group activity with other parents and their children facilitated by an art therapist. Two or three staff members move through the play area observing and providing assistance to parents, and intervening if parental behaviour seems inappropriate. There are several small areas where the parents can sit and talk with their children separately and read or listen to music with them. Outside, there is a playground where parents can play more actively with their children. In addition to these recreational opportunities, brief family therapy sessions are made available and there is a group for biological parents to share their problems with the agency, and discuss their parenting needs.

A similar service, known as the Family Connection Center has also been described by Hess et al. (1992). Like the Family Reunification Program, this service offers transportation to the agency where supervised on-site visits are scheduled between biological parents and their children. The service is provided on a fee-for-service basis to the statutory child protection agency. Although no data were provided, Hess et al. claimed that the service improved the frequency and reliability of parental visiting.

Agency practice has been found to be strongly associated with parental visiting. Reviewing the case records of 256 randomly selected children in care, Proch and Howard (1986) found that most parents tended to comply with visiting schedules drawn up by the social worker. Where there was no plan, or where parents were advised to request visits, visiting did not take place. Plans were not individualized or changed to accommodate changing family circumstances, and they seemed more suited to agency and social worker convenience than to the needs of the children and parents.

In her study of 221 cases in one administrative region of the South Australian statutory authority, Drury-Hudson (1995) identified various agency factors affecting parent–child visiting. The social workers surveyed felt that they needed better resources; more training for themselves, carers and community aides; better review procedures; clearer guidelines, practice standards and policy; and better liaison with fostering agencies. While it was established that 20 per cent of the children were not receiving access visits, the reason given for 42 per cent of these cases was merely that 'the child had been in long-term foster care for some time and access had not occurred' (p. 19). Apart from begging the question, this 'reason' seems to suggest a certain resignation on the part of social workers that visits will inevitably cease over time. For a further 21 per cent of cases, no reason was specified. In 22 per cent of cases it was stated that parents had not initiated or kept access appointments and in 13 per cent of cases the parent or foster carer had moved interstate. In only 1 per cent of cases had the court ordered that access should not take place, and in a further 1 per cent the child did not want contact.

In an Irish study by Gilligan (1996), the foster carer's perspective on parent–child contact was obtained in a postal survey of 73 foster carers. More than a third (36.1 per cent) of all respondents questioned whether contact with biological parents was worth the effort and that number rose to almost two-thirds for long-term foster carers. Three-quarters of this group said that they would be very upset if the child were returned to biological parents. Gilligan points out that such ambivalence towards parent–child contact is unhelpful, as younger children leaving care will be returning to parental care and older children moving to independent living may gravitate towards their biological families. It should be noted in passing that the response rate of 54.4 per cent does cast doubt on the representativeness of the sample in this survey.

Through interviews with 20 female foster carers, Miedema and Nason-Clark (1997) established that, although carers recognized the importance of parents to children, the relationship between carers and natural parents was 'at best ... uncomfortable, emotional and rocky; at worst, it was hostile' (p. 22). Carers were protective of the child and felt they had failed the child when parental contact took place. Some feared for the child's safety if parents had a history of violence, they were distressed at the child's behaviour and extra demands after contact, and wanted as little contact with parents as possible. All but one respondent believed that parent–child contact was one of the most problematic areas of fostering.

Foster carers' views on parent–child contact were also revealed in a qualitative retrospective study conducted by Aldgate and Hawley (1986). The authors interviewed 11 foster families to determine factors which had led to placement breakdown. Carers identified ill-defined access between child and biological family as an important factor contributing to breakdown. Another small qualitative study of parent–child contact sought the views of parents, as well as foster carers and professionals in a Therapeutic Foster Care programme (Jivanjee 1999). There was a discrepancy between professionals' belief in the benefits of family contact and their efforts to facilitate contact, notably because of the demands of high case loads. Further, foster carer training did not always include working with biological family, and negative attitudes towards families on the part of both foster carers and professionals were shown to influence practice. As the sample was small and possibly unrepresentative, these findings have limited external validity. However, Cautley and Aldridge (1975) found that, although carers may have been upset by the behaviour of biological family members, this did not generally interfere with the care they gave the child.

In summary, then, regular parental visiting is a highly valued objective of foster care policy and is encouraged wherever possible. In Australia, it is not uncommon for judges to insist that social workers should present the court with parental contact plans and to hold workers accountable for ensuring that the plans are adhered to. As we have seen, the justification for this policy is built on psychological considerations and on the association between parental visiting and timely reunification. In Chapter 9, we will consider the evidence within our own sample for these justifications.

Group treatment for separation distress

Palmer (1990) has reminded social workers that separation from one's family is almost always a traumatic experience and that children entering foster care therefore need assistance in adjusting to the separation. She describes a structured group programme in which foster children from different foster homes come together to share their experiences and their reactions to separation from biological parents. In the first session, children are prompted to talk about their separation experiences by an eight-item questionnaire seeking their opinions about how separation should be handled. In the second session, a 'Life History Grid' is used to encourage participants to graph significant life events. Subsequent sessions then build on issues raised in the two opening sessions. Although she did not present any controlled research into her group intervention, Palmer claimed a positive reaction to her intervention from children and their social workers.

Mellor and Storer (1988) reported on group work with foster children aged nine to thirteen with a history of abuse or neglect. The aim of the sessions was to provide a forum for the children to talk about their experiences and to learn that they were not alone in grappling with a range of difficult emotions. There were only seven participants, only four sessions were conducted and no measures were taken, but the researchers nevertheless concluded that the groups had been beneficial in that the children spoke freely about their history and feelings and also made new friendships.

Carer support

Fostering can undoubtedly be a rewarding experience but it is just as certainly a demanding one. There is intuitive sense, therefore, in the suggestion that practical and emotional support should help carers to persist when the going inevitably gets tough. A 1990 US survey of over thirty-five thousand current and former carers was reviewed by Orme, Buehler and Rhodes (cited in Casey Family Program 2000). All carers ranked their reasons either for leaving the system (former carers) or for potentially leaving in the future (current carers). Of current carers planning to leave, 46 per cent said that not having a say in the child's future would be their main reason for leaving, 46 per cent also cited difficulty in seeing the child leave, and 36 per cent cited lack of agency support. Reasons given by former carers were lack of agency support (40 per cent), poor communication with the worker (38 per cent), and the child's behaviour (36 per cent).

Despite the apparent importance of agency support for carer persistence, Bebbington and Miles (1990) object that there is very little solid evidence to support any association between carer support and placement outcome. Indeed, results of one Canadian study imply that carer support may contribute very little. This Foster Care Research Project (Steinhauer *et al.* 1989) was a prospective study which compared two models of foster care support. The study randomly assigned carers to a traditional, individual support condition and a group support condition which was jointly run by an experienced foster care couple and a social worker. The group provided guidance and support and performed most of the functions usually assumed by individual caseworkers. Group meetings were held twice a week for two hours throughout the two years of the project. The two experimental conditions were compared on measures of foster parent satisfaction, rate of placement breakdown, carer retention, emotional disturbance in foster children and referrals for residential placement. Results indicated only one significant difference between conditions – foster carers in the group condition felt more supported in their work than did carers assigned to individual social workers.

On the other hand, numerous other authors have, with varying degrees of empirical support, claimed a link between support and placement success or failure (Macaskill 1991), carer retention (Jones 1975; Rowe, Hundleby and Garnett 1989), and placement breakdown (Berridge and Cleaver 1987; Cliffe and Berridge 1991). For example, the views of UK foster carers on the qualities they seek in social workers were obtained via a postal survey (Fisher *et al.* 2000). The 487 respondents were representative of the population of carers in respect of most social characteristics, and the sex and age distributions of the children in their care were in keeping with national figures. Carers wanted support from social workers; specifically they wanted them to show an interest, to listen, to keep them informed and included in planning, and to involve them where appropriate.

A postal survey of 539 carers in the USA (Denby, Rindfleisch and Bean 1999) produced similar findings: that carers want approval, support, timely responses and information, and to have their skills recognized and utilized. And Gilbertson and Barber (in press) recently gathered information about what kinds of support carers want via in-depth interviews with 19 carers who had recently terminated placements on the grounds of the young person's difficult behaviour. Despite the fact that most of the young people involved had displayed extremes of behaviour, such as property damage, assault, theft, truancy, running away, etc., almost half of the carers reported that they would have maintained the placement if a prompt and appropriate crisis response service had been provided, and if they had not been excluded from decision-making about the child.

A recent study by Nixon (1997) suggests that support can be a broad concept. A questionnaire was administered to sixty-seven foster carers followed by a semi-structured interview schedule to a sub-group of twenty of these same carers. An important limitation of this study is that all of the carers involved had been the subject of an unsubstantiated allegation of abusing the child in their care. This limitation notwithstanding, social worker support was of value only to a minority of the carers at times of such crisis. Results suggested that carers' choice of support was a very personal one which was dependent on a number of factors, such as the degree of support they felt within their own informal support networks.

The importance of informal support networks was also demonstrated by a comprehensive foster carer training programme developed in Canada and run in several communities (Titterington 1990). Agencies working with children in care participated, and the training programme was constructed to encourage a team approach, networking and full use of community resources, as well as to provide general carer training. Data on networking were obtained at baseline and after programme completion. Analysis of contacts showed that carers had a variety of frequent and positive contacts but that they were most often in touch with friends, relatives and neighbours and least often with social services staff. Informal contacts were said to be supportive, whereas formal contacts were instrumental. In general, training resulted in more contact with other foster carers and a decrease in contact with social workers.

In their small study of 12 foster families caring for sexually abused children, Henry et al. (1991) reported that social workers and foster carers typically disagree about the amount of training and support carers receive. More specifically, the majority of carers in their study indicated that they would have liked to receive more services such as education on sexual abuse, child development and behaviour management training. A significant minority of the sample also expressed a need to participate in support groups for foster parents. The most likely explanation for the inconsistency in studies of carer support is that outcomes are associated with specific kinds or schedules of support, and not just any form of support will do. The practice implication of these findings would appear to be that, while carers want support and can specify the types of support they need, it may not be provided best by agency staff under all circumstances. As a result, the adequacy of both formal *and* informal support systems needs to be addressed.

Carer remuneration

It is widely believed that the rate of payment to foster carers has little or nothing to do with the decision to foster or to persist with fostering. No doubt this perception is largely attributable to the self-reports of carers themselves, who rarely mention payment among their list of motives. Rather, they tend to emphasize altruistic motives and their love of children (Department of Family and Community Services 1997). For example, Miedema and Nason-Clark (1997), in a qualitative study involving female foster carers, found a reluctance on the part of carers to see themselves as professionals. The researchers were interested in the attitude of foster carers to professionalization following the restructure of foster care services in New Brunswick, Canada. The restructure involved categorizing care provision at four distinct levels with remuneration according to level and promotion dependent upon completion of mandatory training and, at the highest level, teaching parenting skills to biological families. This restructure was intended to address the shortage of foster families and to operationalize an inclusive model of foster care. However, the respondents saw fostering as an extension of mothering and a labour of love, and rejected notions of themselves as counsellors, therapists or teachers. Smith (1988) also found carer ambivalence in respect of fostering as both 'labour' and 'love' and a reluctance on the part of carers to consider reimbursement for 'mothering' which, even if required as work, they find intrinsically rewarding. Butler and Charles (1999) conducted a small qualitative study of carers and young people who had experienced placement breakdown. One of the problems they identified was that payment to carers inhibited the young person's ability to see their carer as a parental figure and therefore to sustain appropriate relationships with her. For both carers and young people, payment seemed to be at odds with societal values about parenting and love.

Despite such findings, research by Campbell and Downs (1987) shows that both recruitment and retention of foster carers are actually quite sensitive to variations in price. The results of multiple regression analysis of data from over a thousand foster families across eight US states showed that the supply of foster carers was significantly associated with a measure of the 'real board rate' accruing to the child. Results of this study are consistent with a more recent survey of current and former non-relative carers conducted throughout the United States by Rhodes, Orme and Buehler (2001), who found inadequate reimbursement to be high among carers' reasons for leaving the system. And in a randomized, controlled study, Chamberlain, Moreland and Reid (1992) investigated the effect of increased support and stipend. Foster carers were assigned to one of three conditions: enhanced support and training plus increased payment; increased payment only; or standard foster care without enhanced training or increased payment. Carers were assessed within the first three weeks of placement, then three, six and nine months later. Foster carer drop-out rates were 9.6 per cent for the enhanced training and payment group, 14.3 per cent for the increased payment only group and 25.9 per cent for the control group. Further, more children with carers in the enhanced training and payment group had significantly more successful days in care than children with carers in the other two groups.

External case review

While periodic case review is routine in most jurisdictions, few foster care programmes make use of external reviewers. Among those that have is a citizen-judicial review process described by Wert, Fein and Haller (1986). In this programme, volunteer reviewers attend all formal case reviews and court hearings. Depending upon whether or not court-determined expectations are being met, volunteers may request an earlier judicial review. In this study, cases subject to the review process were compared with cases from before its implementation. The median length of time for which cases were open and awaiting disposition was twenty-two weeks prior to citizen-judicial review and twelve weeks following its introduction. And in the USA, the child welfare agency in the District of Columbia contracted independent professionals to review cases. Children and parents were also encouraged to participate in the review, and private and public agency staff responded to a survey questionnaire to evaluate the process. The majority of the 75 respondents said that the reviews were helpful and identified higher rates of family participation and reunification as benefits to flow from the review system (Leashore 1986).

Jennings, McDonald and Henderson (1996) randomly allocated 46 'children-in-need-of-care' cases to early (within 45 days of a child entering the system) citizen case review and 39 cases to a control condition. The children were followed up at three-monthly intervals and, although results were not statistically significant, the authors claimed that there was a consistent trend in favour of early citizen review. Review cases were less likely to seek extensions of court orders and social workers reported that the reviews had caused them to recognize problems with renewals that they otherwise would have missed. In addition, more services were mobilized for the review cases early in the life of the case, and more services were needed later in the life of control cases. The authors also reported that review cases were more likely to have a written case plan containing clearly specified goals. Finally, a smaller percentage of children in the review group experienced multiple placements, although there was no difference between groups in the percentage of reunified cases at the final follow-up point.

Leaving care

In Australia, most children and young people leave foster care in one of two ways: either they return to their family of origin or they move to independent living. In recent years, there has been a move towards conceiving of reunification as a process rather than an event. Reunification can occur at any point on a continuum of outcomes from parent–child contact to the full restoration of the child to the family system (Maluccio, Warsh and Pine 1993). It must be said, though, that the reunification literature almost invariably deals with reunification as full restoration of the child to the family of origin.

It is known that reunification is unsuccessful for a substantial minority of children and that, with each re-entry to care, the likelihood of successful reunification decreases (Bullock, Little and Millham 1993; Farmer 1993). Maluccio, Fein and Davis (1994) reviewed studies on re-entry to care and found that reported rates ranged from 10 per cent to 33 per cent. Rzepnicki (1987) also reviewed the literature on recidivism of children who had been returned to their parents after a spell in foster care, or who had gone to another form of placement intended to be permanent. She found rates of 20–30 per cent, with the highest rates being for children who were returned to their families of origin. Family-of-origin factors associated with recidivism in this study included the child's behaviour problems and parents' inability to control the behaviour, inadequate parenting skills, parents' having requested the initial placement and inadequate housing and/or income. Similarly, Festinger (1994) found that family-of-origin factors featured prominently among reasons for re-entry to care in her study of 210 children aged under fifteen years who were discharged home from a spell in foster care of sixty days or longer. Twenty-seven (12.9 per cent) returned to care within twelve months of discharge. Reasons most frequently cited were alcohol or substance abuse, abuse of the child, parenting difficulties and the child's unmanageable behaviour.

Farmer (1993) stresses that return home must be understood and managed as a major transition which necessitates renegotiation of the child's roles and relationships in the home and other settings in which they are involved. She points out that many children return to families that have changed in circumstances or composition since entry to care, and families may have assumed a new way of functioning which does not include the child. Bullock, Little and Millham (1993) see return home as a series of episodes: changes in family circumstances, return home becomes an issue, return home, honeymoon period, acrimonious negotiations between family members and the establishment of a new *modus vivendi*.

The most prominent intervention in the area of family reunification is family preservation services. Features of this model include time-limited in-home services, provision of material services and the availability of twenty-four-hour emergency assistance. Services are said to be based upon family empowerment and the belief that children are best raised by their own family (Pecora *et al.* 1987). In a study of the application of the Intensive Family Preservation Services (IFPS) model to reunification, Gillespie, Byrne and

Workman (1995) conducted a pilot study of forty-two children in state custody whose biological and foster families participated in a reunification project. Inclusion criteria were the biological family's availability and willingness to receive project services. Exclusion criteria were sexual abuse cases judged to require long-term intervention, and cases of severe physical abuse. In a quasi-experimental design, IFPS services (including in-home therapy, parent education and liaison with community agencies) were supplemented by enhanced parent–child visiting, specialized carer training, enhanced worker contact with carers and linking of foster and biological families. At the end of the intervention (the median duration of service was six months), 33 children had returned to parents or relatives. At one-year follow-up, 91 per cent of the reunified children remained at home. Perhaps not surprisingly, there was a strong association between reunification and the mother's attitude to the child's return home. Twenty-eight of the 30 children whose mothers were positive about reunification were returned home, compared with 5 of the 12 children whose mothers were ambivalent about reunification.

Bullock, Little and Millham's (1993) large study of children returned to their families after a spell in foster care identified several factors that were associated with successful reunification. These include: first return home, the child not being an offender, high-quality family relationships and preparation of the family for the return. Highly competent social work was also shown to be associated with successful reunification: specifically this involved a case plan that kept the family involved and was tailored to the family's time-frames. It also included social workers making themselves available when needed and having confidence in and being committed to reunification. Farmer (1993) also found that effective social work was important to successful reunification. She compared outcomes for unallocated cases with those which had continuous social work involvement during return home and found that the latter were significantly more likely to be successful. Specific social work practices associated with positive outcomes were: decisive planning for the child's return, the social worker maintaining initiative for the return, the child's progress being monitored, the risk level being clearly recorded, parental involvement in six-monthly reviews and enforcement of conditions associated with reunification.

The need to prepare adolescents in foster care for independent living has also been well documented (English, Kouidou-Giles and Plocke 1994; Mech, Ludy-Dobson and Hulseman 1994). The move from foster care to independent living is increasingly being recognized and managed as a process rather than an event (Cunningham and Freeman 1993), and many advocate services that approximate the support that parents provide for children moving to independent living (Cunningham and Freeman 1993; Taylor 1990). Mendes and Goddard (2000) contrast the abrupt transition to independence traditionally expected of young people leaving foster care with the long and supported transition period normally experienced by young people leaving their biological family. A recent Australian study (Maunders *et al.* 1999) into the circumstances of young people leaving care found that, although governments have recognized the need for preparation for independent living and initiated some programmes, much remains to be done to support young people before, during and after leaving care. Among the problems impeding the transition to independence are unstable post-care accommodation, inadequate income, contact with the justice system, pregnancy soon after leaving care and lack of ongoing contact with the care system. Conversely, a stable and positive experience of care, availability of mentors or advocates, continuing support by carers and social workers, and family contact while in care, were all found to promote successful transition to independence.

Mallon (1992) makes the point that, for children under the age of thirteen years whose lives have been sufficiently disrupted to require foster care, there is often a need to provide training in basic life skills. The so-called Junior Life Skills curriculum he developed consists of eighteen units of 109 life skills lessons designed as an aid for foster carers and child care workers. The programme takes nothing for granted and covers very basic skills such as brushing one's teeth. Each unit consists of several lessons embodying objectives, methods, materials and suggested activities.

For older children, the focus of living skills programmes needs to be on training for the transition to independence. Adolescent programmes in the United States, for example, typically consist of training in both 'hard' skills such as money management and cooking, and 'soft' skills such as building social support networks (McMillen *et al.* 1997). While evaluations of these programmes generally report positive results (e.g. Mech and Rycroft 1995; Scannapieco, Schagrin and Scannapieco 1995), the successful components are not always clearly identified, and small sample size and lack of control groups limit the usefulness of findings (e.g. Mallon 1998).

As Hahn (1994) pointed out, not all young people in care need all services, and assessment must be a fundamental component of any independent living programme. In his study of sixteen- to nineteen-year-olds in care, he found that between one-fifth and one-third of those tested were in need of specialized services as well as follow-up and/or aftercare. Stone (1989) conducted a survey of leaving care schemes in the UK. Interviews with 32 care leavers showed that the most frequently used services were advice, information, accommodation, preparation for leaving care training, and volunteer help and support. Services nominated by respondents as being most needed in order of priority were: financial help, a range of accommodation options, education and training or practical help and support, advice and information, and counselling.

Maunders and colleagues (1999) studied leaving care via a convenience sample recruited through agencies across mainland Australia. Of the 37 respondents, 18 had received some preparation for leaving care, including independent living programmes, but 11 of the 18 said that despite this they had been inadequately prepared. Young people were discharged from the age of sixteen, yet more than two-thirds of them had not been involved in any discussion about discharge. Not surprisingly, then, discharge for some is experienced as an abrupt process involving sudden and complete cessation of contact with care systems. Foster care agencies typically have limited resources for young people after discharge, allocation is discretionary and services are often inadequate. While some young people were happy to be discharged, most found sudden independence difficult to manage and described reactions such as depression, fear, turning to drugs or alcohol, loneliness, and feeling rejected.

Ryan *et al.* (1988) suggest that foster carers are best placed to teach living skills to the young people in their care but that carers are an under-utilized resource in this area. Because they are in daily contact with the young person, carers are able to take advantage of learning opportunities as they arise. Further, they are aware of the areas in which the young person has skill deficits and this enables them to provide a learning programme specific to the young person's needs. The authors note that as a prerequisite to teaching living skills, carers require training in adolescent development, the effects of abuse and neglect on development, adolescent sexuality, and loss and grief reactions, as well as the skills to assess deficits. They must also be able to negotiate difficult areas such as providing structure and security for the young person while also providing the flexibility and freedom to make mistakes and learn from them.

Summary

As was the case for the literature dealing with assessment and planning, empirically valid generalizations are difficult to make about the characteristics of optimal placements and transition from care. Among the less contentious propositions that can be extracted from the literature are the following:

- External case reviews expedite case plans.
- Most foster children prefer sibling co-placement.
- Kinship care is associated with higher levels of contact between foster children and their biological families.
- Kinship care is associated with fewer placement moves.
- In the United States, kinship care is associated with lower rates of biological family reunification.
- Kinship foster care is associated with lower levels of access to support systems.
- Most foster children want to maintain contact with their biological parents.
- Parental visits decline in frequency and reliability over time.

The best supported family-based option for behaviourally and emotionally troubled adolescents is Treatment Foster Care (TFC). The most important characteristics of TFC include:

- Carers are chosen specifically to deal with the most difficult children in care.
- Carers receive a higher rate of payment than standard foster carers.
- Carers are contracted as employees by the relevant agency.
- Carers are actively involved in case planning as full and equal members of the team.
- Carers undergo longer and more intensive training than do regular foster carers.
- Carers receive ongoing in-service training.
- Normally only one child is assigned to a TFC carer at a time.
- The case load of the agency support worker is reduced to enable extra support for carers.

Other empirically supported propositions include:

- Carer support programmes that make use of the carer's informal support networks are associated with better placement outcomes.
- The best predictors of carer retention are: (1) rate of remuneration, and (2) carer reliance on the income from foster care.
- The transition to independent living is facilitated by training in living skills and the provision of material services such as financial aid, accommodation and job training.

Our review of the extant literature has also identified a number of promising developments in the foster care field that are worthy of further investigation. Among these are:

- Parental visiting centres where children and their biological parents can meet and relax with one another, and where children's groups and biological parents' groups can be conducted.
- Group sessions for children during their transition to care to ease anxiety and to ameliorate loss and grief.

As well as the need for caution about the supporting evidence for much of what is currently thought to represent best practice in foster care, it is very important to recognize the need to tailor our methods to the particular needs of the foster child. There is a tendency in much of the literature to conceive of foster care as a single service rather than as a generic term for a range of potential placement options occurring within a family setting. To the extent that this view prevails in practice, it runs the risk of ignoring individual differences in foster children and of stifling the development of creative approaches to the care of sub-groups within the foster care population. As we will show in later chapters, one particularly disadvantaged group of children in care comprises emotionally or behaviourally troubled children for whom highly intensive, individualized foster placements are likely to be necessary.

Part II

Background to the study

Chapter 3

From parent to purchaser

The new policy context

Introduction

Throughout the western world, family-based foster care is facing similar challenges, to which most governments are responding in broadly similar ways. Among the most important of these challenges are declining numbers of carers coupled with growing numbers of children who are displaying more serious and intractable problems than was the case even a decade or so ago. In the USA, Britain and Australia, one predictable response to the crisis has been 'outsourcing' or devolution of the foster care system to non-government agencies operating under contract to government. In this chapter we describe how these factors came together in South Australia just as our research was getting under way. Because it sets out the policy context of our work, this chapter helps to explain many of the issues and problems our work uncovered. Although the details of this outline are necessarily limited to Australia, readers from North America, Britain and continental Europe will no doubt recognize many of the issues within their own countries.

In South Australia, as in all Australian states except New South Wales (see Chapter 1), adoption is not an option for most of the children in alternative care and there is no provision under South Australia's Children's Protection Act 1993 for permanent termination of parental rights, although in extreme cases the court may proscribe contact with certain family members. In most cases, social workers are required to ensure that the child has the best possible connection with their birth family, even in cases where the family has been abusive (Department for Family and Community Services 1996). Although state government ministers are ultimately responsible for providing out-of-home care for children, governments have never worked alone. Throughout Australia, state governments have traditionally provided some out-of-home care placements, but they have also licensed and funded alternative care providers within the non-government sector. Indeed, non-government welfare agencies have been involved in the provision of alternative care services from the very earliest days of white settlement in Australia (Dickey 1980). Prior to the restructuring of foster care services that occurred in South Australia towards the end of 1997, some foster placements were provided by the government department responsible for child welfare (currently called Family and Youth Services (FAYS)), and others were provided by a range of non-government (mainly Church) agencies. In the case of Aboriginal children, there was (and still is) a separate, government-funded unit, staffed by Aboriginal workers, who arrange or ratify all placements. The individuals and families who made their homes available for foster care were (and still are) licensed by the state but were affiliated with one or other of the 'provider' agencies. The support, management and supervision of the carers was the responsibility of the agency concerned. Foster carers have always been volunteer workers in South Australia, so they are compensated rather than remunerated for their work. Both before and after the restructuring of alternative care, the level of compensation to carers has been under the control of the state rather than the foster care agency, and children with high needs or challenging behaviours, for example, attract a loading known as 'special needs loading' in recognition of the higher costs associated with caring for them.

The changing role of the state in community service provision

As with most non-government welfare programmes supported by public funds, budgets for alternative care agencies were essentially 'grants-based' until quite recently. Under the grants-based approach, agencies petition the government for the funds to provide services, and the amount awarded tends to be determined by a combination of service history and the persuasiveness of the agency's submission. The approach is therefore reactive in the sense that it responds to submissions from provider organizations. Not only do the strongest and most articulate organizations tend to receive most of the funding, but the scope for centralized planning and accountability is limited because policy direction is driven more by the service provider than the funder. Service reviews tend to be conducted as part of the latest funding round and are based more on precedent than on demand. Such funding arrangements have the potential to produce a flurry of inappropriate spending as funding reviews loom and providers need to demonstrate that renewed funding is necessary. Government policy-makers these days take the view that the grants-based approach has created inefficiency and duplication in the human services, especially in the administrative and management structures of service providers (see, for example, Lee 1987).

The movement away from grants-based funding towards contestability is also consistent with a microeconomic reform agenda that has been vigorously pursued in Australia for decades now. The fundamental objective of the agenda has been to increase competitiveness of the Australian economy, and this has so far taken three main forms. The first is deregulation or the systematic removal of government legislation that inhibits or controls business practices. The second is corporatization or the introduction of private-sector management styles into the public sector. The third is privatization or the sale of government-owned businesses or assets into private share holdings. In 1992, the then Keating Labor government established the Hilmer Committee of Inquiry into competition policy in Australia (Hilmer, Reyner and Tapperell 1993). Following the Hilmer Report, Federal Parliament passed the Competition Policy Reform Act 1995, modifying the Trade Practices Act in line with the Hilmer Committee's recommendations. Some have argued (e.g. Quiggin 1998) that this Act was the most significant legacy of the Keating Labor government. The Act bound both state and federal governments to implement comprehensive pro-market reforms, to be overseen by a National Competition Council. The most noteworthy examples are the corporatization of government business enterprises and a comprehensive programme of competitive tendering and contracting for publicly provided services.

Through the microeconomic reform process, Australian governments have been tacitly redefining the role they wish to play in society. In particular, the acceptance by governments of the principles outlined in Australia's national competition policy has promoted a minimalist approach to government intervention. An increasing number of community services are being contracted out to private providers, and public sector reforms have as explicit objectives cutbacks in funding and staffing levels. In essence, Australian governments are reconstructing themselves as 'purchasers' rather than 'providers' of public services. Under this approach, the funder (the Ministers and their advisers) establishes the broad directions and framework for the service. The funder then allocates a budget to the purchaser, who has responsibility for obtaining specific outcomes or 'deliverables' at the best available price. In order to apply the model, functioning markets and competition need to exist, so the model seeks to integrate human services into a part of the service market – the so-called quasi-market. Through competition and the closer alignment of service delivery with the needs of consumers, the state positions itself as the customer among a number of potential suppliers. According to its proponents, the model promotes clearer service definition, greater accountability and an objective framework for priority resolution (Family and Community Services 1995). The Industry Commission (1997) captured the essence of the new approach to community services in this way:

Relationships with external providers of human services

Grants based funding relationships are typically characterised by:

- competition for funds through informal processes
- few, if any, explicit performance or output measures
- one-off or annual funding commitments

- renewal of funding based on the previous year's expenditure, and
- service characteristics and access criteria not being explicit.

Purchase of service relationships are typically characterised by:

- more explicitly defined selection criteria for providers which can include price and/or quality
- explicit performance measures
- multiple year contracts
- renewal of funding based on re-examination of client needs and service costs
- the purchaser specifying the service characteristics and access criteria.

Not surprisingly, the purchaser-provider model of statutory service provision has had quite fundamental implications for the relationship between government and non-government agencies and for relations within the sector as a whole. Taking their ideological lead from Margaret Thatcher's Britain, Australian government departments no longer conceive of themselves as partners with the community sector but as brokers of public funds whose role is to maximize the return on taxpayers' money through the promotion of competition between potential providers (see, for example, Robbins 1997). The consequences of this shift on working relations in the foster care sector will be discussed in Chapter 5.

The abandonment of residential alternatives to foster care

The emphasis on family preservation that is evident in child welfare policy today is part of a worldwide change in child protection legislation that reasserted the rights of the birth parents. Notwithstanding New South Wales's recent adoption of the American philosophy of permanency planning (see Chapter 1), child welfare policy throughout Australia continues to place strict limits on state intervention and aims to return children to the care of their birth families as soon as possible. When statutory intervention is necessary, state governments prefer informal, community-based approaches such as foster care over residential options. Not only is foster care cheaper but at its best models the kind of nuclear family to which the state aims to return the child.

Figure 3.1 indicates that the population in alternative care nationwide fell from 17,920 in 1983 to 12,273 in 1993. More importantly, the decline in the alternative care population that occurred during that time was almost entirely accounted for by residential care, which used to be the option of choice for children who are difficult to care for in family homes (Fratter *et al.* 1991; Hudson, Nutter and Galaway 1994; Whittaker, Tripodi and

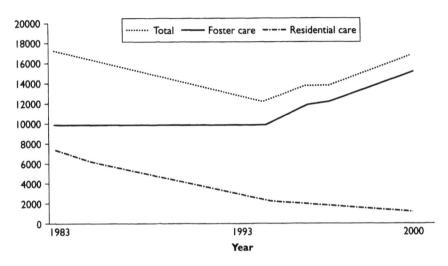

Figure 3.1 Australian population in care

Grasso 1990; Scholte 1997). In 1983 there were 7,410 children in residential care, but that number had fallen to 2,455 by 1993. By contrast, the numbers in foster care remained relatively constant between 1983 and 1993. Figure 3.1 presents another important dimension of the quiet revolution in alternative care policy. In response to mounting public concern about children at risk following the Burdekin Inquiry into Youth Homelessness (Burdekin 1989), and after a series of highly publicized judicial complaints about the parlous state of child protection services in Victoria and New South Wales, the numbers of children taken into foster care, but not residential care, began to rise after 1993. By the year 2000, the numbers in alternative care had returned to 1983 levels, entirely as a result of the rapid increase in the number of children entering family-based care (15,169 by the year 2000). Meanwhile, the numbers in residential care continued to fall throughout the period, reaching a mere 1,222 nationwide by the year 2000.

In short, Australia's reliance on foster care has now reached unprecedented levels. As the cheapest out-of-home care option available, foster care is obviously attractive to governments with an eye to cutting their outlays on welfare.

The United States and Britain have also witnessed declines in residential (sometimes called 'group' or 'congregate') care coupled with rapid increases in the use of foster care. By the year 2000, for example, there were around 570,000 American children in foster care, which was more than double the number a decade earlier (US Department of Health and Human Services 2000), despite a federally legislated requirement to move foster children

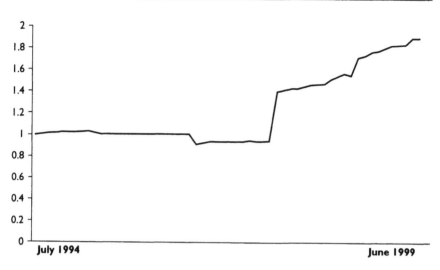

Figure 3.2 Percentage of foster children in receipt of loading

expeditiously towards adoption (see Chapter 1). Meanwhile, the number of children entering group care in the USA has been falling steadily. And in Britain the number of children looked after by local authorities in foster care rose by 16 per cent between 1996 and 2001 while the numbers in residential care fell by 11 per cent over the same period (Department of Health 2002).

Among the more important consequences of this shift away from residential care has been a severe shortage of placements for emotionally disturbed children and adolescents, and for children with disabilities. Throughout the western world, increasingly difficult children are being foisted on reluctant foster parents, resulting in an alarming rate of placement breakdown as volunteer carers discover that they have neither the skills nor the desire to deal with the children they are assigned (Department of Health 2002; Barber, Delfabbro and Cooper 2001). Another consequence of the demise of residential care in Australia is the growing prevalence of 'special needs loadings' which are payable to foster parents for expenses incurred in housing children with special needs such as disability, mental illness or severe emotional or behavioural disorders. Figure 3.2 shows that the proportion of foster parents in receipt of special needs loadings in South Australia, for example, has been rising dramatically in recent years

The collision between demography and social policy

The most fundamental problem with the growing reliance on foster care is that it is entirely at odds with social and demographic forces in western societies today. Perhaps the most important of these is the torrent of women who have entered the workforce over recent decades. In both its scale and its implications for society, the world has witnessed few other movements like it. In Australia, for example, the workforce participation of married women has more than doubled since 1966 (Australian Bureau of Statistics 2002), and working women today make up around 45 per cent (and rising) of all employment. Half of all women with children under the age of five are now in some form of paid employment. This figure rises to around two-thirds by the time the children are between six and twelve and to 80 per cent by the time the children reach high school (Glezer 1991; Kilmartin 1997). With women traditionally filling the role of carer, their increased workforce participation has meant that there is a shrinking pool of volunteers to work as foster parents.

The problem is compounded by the ageing of the populations of western countries, which has meant that working women and men are increasingly called upon to care for elderly relatives. In fact, in this century for the first time in Australia's history, more employees will have dependent elders than dependent children (Gibbs 1996), which will reduce the pool of available carers still further. Meanwhile, the capacity of families to bear the extra burden has diminished in line with the dramatic rise in single-parent households that followed the Family Law Act of 1976. Ever since the Act made divorce an easier and more humane option for Australian couples, the national divorce rate has climbed to its present rate of around 45 per cent (Australian Bureau of Statistics 1999).

Deregulation of the labour market following the Workplace Relations Act 1996 has also played its part in reducing Australia's capacity for voluntary work. The Workplace Relations Act codified a trend that had been occurring in Australia for many years towards reduction in unionization and union power, together with an industrial relations system that encourages enterprise bargains and workplace agreements which do not necessarily flow on to other industries or workplaces. Experience in New Zealand, the United States and Australia under conditions of labour market deregulation indicates that enterprise bargaining increases the burden of work on most families (Barber in press; Gibbs 1996; Maloney 1994; Yeabsley and Savage 1996). For example, a recent Australian study into the effects of deregulation of working hours (Charlesworth 1996) showed that the much-vaunted flexibility of enterprise bargaining often works against the interests of female workers with family responsibilities by forcing those in service industries to work longer hours and irregular shifts.

Putting these social forces together with the policy drift towards foster care, it is apparent that current out-of-home care policy simply cannot be reconciled with the social and demographic realities of life in Australia today. Figure 3.3 illustrates the point with South Australian data, but the same situation applies all over the country.

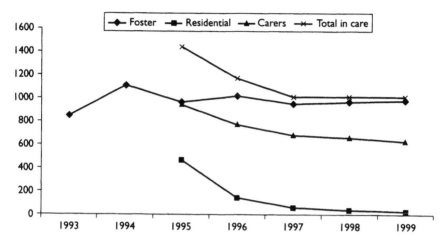

Figure 3.3 Demand for care and availability of carers

Figure 3.3 presents the total number of South Australian children in care between 30 June 1995 and 30 June 1999. It also records the number of children in residential care over the same period, as well as the numbers in foster care and the number of carers available to care for them. It shows clearly that the gap between demand for and supply of foster carers has been widening. The trajectories of these lines have not changed since that time. Meanwhile, the number of children in residential care fell every year for which reliable data are available, from a high of 441 in 1995 to a mere 36 in 1999. Similarly, in the USA between 1986 and 1996, the number of children in foster care rose by around 90 per cent, while the number of available carers fell by 3 per cent. This situation is obviously unsustainable. Even if the growth in foster care levels out in the years ahead, the decline in available carers will continue.

South Australia's restructured alternative care system

In South Australia, an internal Family and Community Services (FACS) review of alternative care services was conducted in 1992 as the gaps in the system continued to widen (Dini and Olivieri 1993). The review was timely because the impending introduction of the Children's Protection Act 1993 had significant implications for all of FACS' services, including alternative care. Under the Act, intervention by the state when dealing with a child has to be the least disruptive and should aim to maintain the child in a familiar environment. Thus, it was clear that the new legislation would place additional demand on short-term placements and put pressure on alternative care providers to step up their family reunification efforts. In particular, there would be a need to recruit greater numbers of foster families willing to work intensively with birth families to facilitate reunification. It was also expected that the Act would produce an increase in relative (or 'kinship') care.

Among the major findings of the Foster Care Services review was that there was an urgent shortage of foster carers within non-government agencies despite some of them making valiant recruitment efforts (Dini and Olivieri 1993). The situation was particularly acute in the rural areas. In addition to placement shortages, the review commented on inefficiencies in the system resulting from there being too many providers with rigid barriers to co-operation between them. In the authors' view, this lack of co-operation was responsible for unnecessary duplication especially in recruitment and training. The authors also felt that exclusive ownership of carers by the different agencies was an obstacle to matching children and carers because the most suitable carer for any given child was not necessarily to be found within the agency to which the child was assigned.

In the area of service costs, Dini and Olivieri (1993) noted that FACS supported between 61 per cent and 71 per cent of foster care placements with only 38 per cent of dedicated staffing resources. While commenting on the apparently lower unit cost of government compared with non-government foster care, the authors were careful not to conclude that the government sector was more cost-effective for the obvious reason that their study contained no measures of service quality or outcome. Setting aside also the fact that the authors took no account of non-staffing costs, economies of scale and administrative efficiencies, all of which worked in favour of FACS, it was nevertheless apparent that, unless the total amount of money in the system was increased, any successful tenderer from the non-government sector would have to settle for considerably less funding per child after taking over FACS' part of the service.

On the basis of their research, Dini and Olivieri (1993) made a number of recommendations in addition to the need to avoid duplication of services and to remove barriers between agencies. The authors also pointed to the need for FACS workers to involve foster carers in decisions about the child, the need for better information systems, more placements and a greater range of placement options. Finally, the authors suggested that the increased demand on foster care services should be met through increased productivity rather than by increased funding.

A separate internal review (Denley and Wilson 1993) found even more pressing problems in foster care services for children with disabilities. This review was a joint project of FACS and the Intellectual Disability Services Council (IDSC) to examine the placement needs of children with disabilities, and the provision and management of these placements. It was undertaken largely because of administrative problems surrounding children with disabilities in the alternative care system. At the heart of these problems was the fact that for clients of IDSC to gain access to out-of-home placements, they had to be referred to FACS. According to the authors of the report (Denley and Wilson 1993) this situation had created 'considerable tension' (p. 10) between FACS and IDSC because it was unclear which agency had responsibility for what aspects of the case.

The authors found, as had another review three years earlier (Cross 1990), that the service system for children with disabilities and their families was in crisis, primarily because of the closure of residential facilities in pursuit of a policy of 'deinstitutionalizing' children to 'the community'. Among the services urgently needed were:

- emergency and respite care, especially in country areas
- out-of-school-hours care for children of working parents
- intensive behaviour management programmes
- in-home family support in the form of practical home assistance and childcare
- non-English-speaking services
- long-term accommodation, particularly for children of elderly parents
- intensive family support at times of crisis
- foster care
- residential care generally.

The review concluded that the entire area of substitute care for children with disabilities was under-resourced and that additional services had to be created urgently. The authors recommended the establishment of a specialized disability foster care agency because the operational processes and procedures in the field were so deficient. There was, for instance, little clarity or consistency in the division of responsibilities between FACS and IDSC. The two agencies passed responsibility back and forth, and both complained that they were not resourced to provide the service. Meanwhile, families were provided with contradictory advice and an inadequate level of service.

Amongst other things, these internal reviews showed that the pressures on foster care identified earlier in this chapter were already straining foster care to the limit years before FACS decided to restructure its service. The departmental response to the reviews was to establish a Ministerial Reference Group in April 1994. Membership of the Reference Group was drawn from the government and non-government sectors and their terms of reference were to:

1 consider the Foster Care Review (Dini and Olivieri 1993) and the report on Children with Disability Unable to Live at Home (Denley and Wilson 1993) and expand on the options or recommendations presented in the reports

2   advise the Minister regarding the future directions of foster care service delivery in South Australia, with particular reference to current government policy, which would include children with disability.

The Reference Group confirmed the existence of significant problems in South Australia's alternative care system. According to the Reference Group, the most serious of these was the severe shortage of placements, particularly for the following groups:

- emotionally disturbed children and adolescents
- adolescents generally, including those with difficult behaviour problems or mental illness
- children with severe disabilities
- children in transition to adulthood.

Since almost all of the more than a thousand children in alternative care at that time could be placed in one or other of these categories, it is not surprising that the report also identified high rates of multiple placements and numerous reports of children who could not be placed at all.

The Substitute Care Reference Group recommended a complete restructure of the system to be undertaken over three years. Among the list of recommendations were that:

- resources should be directed to services that strengthened families and assisted them to meet their responsibilities towards their children. Such services should include 'a creative respite package' (Substitute Care Reference Group 1994, p. 10) to assist families to care for the child while providing access to out-of-home respite.
- contact between birth parents and their children should be promoted. This recommendation was based on international experience demonstrating that, when family contact is promoted, the odds of placement breakdown are diminished and the likelihood of family reunification enhanced.
- a comprehensive information and database should be developed to facilitate evaluation of service outcomes and outputs.
- alternatives to foster care should be 'seriously considered in the future' (Substitute Care Reference Group 1994, p. 11). According to the Reference Group, there was 'increasing recognition' that foster care was not a viable option for 'a number' of children in the alternative care system. This was because the demands imposed on foster carers by these children were so great that placement breakdown and therefore multiple placements were likely. The Reference Group went on to recommend establishing small, supervised community homes to complement foster care.
- professional family care should also be considered as another alternative to foster care for severely disabled or disturbed children and adolescents.

Finally, the Reference Group further recommended that a government policy for substitute care should be developed which reflected the principles of the new Act and government policy on the provision of public services.

In their final report, Dini and Olivieri (1993) pointed out that the combination of 'non existent overall planning' and 'inadequate communication' had driven foster care programmes apart and led to poor co-ordination and communication between services. (It is most ironic, then, that one of the service providers' major objections to the restructured system is that it has destroyed all co-operation between them as they compete with one another for the funding to mount their services.) The subsequent restructure of alternative care in South Australia can be expressed as in Figure 3.4. As this indicates, the Policy and Development Division, under the Minister, assumed the role of funder, with specific responsibility for strategic policy development and evaluation of the system as a whole. The Community Services Division became the purchaser, responsible for the planning, purchasing and monitoring of services from the non-government sector, and also for managing service contracts. Finally, FACS' Field Services Division was placed in the curious position of being a service provider to the organization of which it was a part, although its responsibility for foster care was to be outsourced as soon as the process of competitive tendering was complete.

Under the new FACS structure, District Centres (the offices of Field Services Division where the day-to-day casework is conducted) were to be the gateway to all out-of-home placements, except for a small number of emergency placements. After outsourcing foster care, District Centres were to refer all out-of-home care requests to FACS' new Central Alternative Care Unit (CACU) which would process the application and refer it in turn to the non-government foster care providers or to one of FACS' residential care units if institutional care was necessary.

Following Ministerial sign-off of the new policy, responsibility for the second stage of the restructure passed to the purchaser (Community Services Division) for the development of a funding plan, and to Field Services Division to commence their own internal planning for the transfer of responsibilities outlined in the policy. The Services and Funding Plan developed by the Community Services Division provided for the outsourcing, through competitive tender, of out-of-home care for children. Tenders were to be restricted to not-for-profit community organizations, effectively limiting competition to the agencies that had previously provided foster care services under grants from FACS.

The core elements of the new service system are four geographically based area services, an Aboriginal service (responsibility for which was to remain with the Aboriginal Child Care Agency, now called Aboriginal Family Services) and a statewide disability service. The area services encompass two metropolitan and two country area services providing emergency, respite, short-term and long-term care within their geographical boundaries. Area

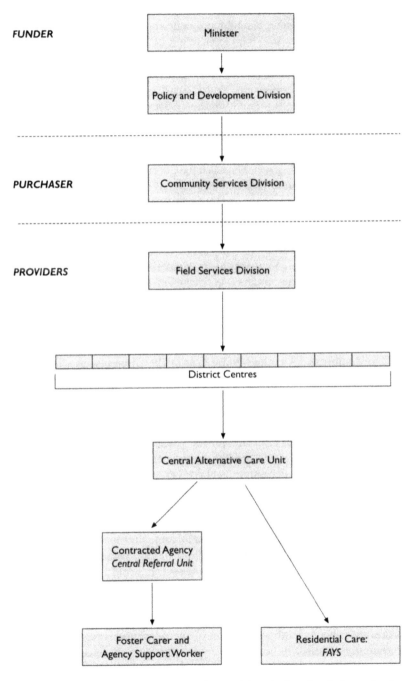

Figure 3.4 The funder–purchaser–provider model applied to South Australia alternative care

services (sometimes also called 'contracted agencies') are now responsible for the recruitment, assessment, training and ongoing support of foster carers.

Since the initial restructuring, the Department of Family and Community Services has been incorporated within a mega-department known as the Department of Human Services (DHS). The Field Services Division of FACS is now the Division of Family and Youth Services (FAYS) within DHS. The Policy and Development, and Community Services Divisions of FACS have also had name changes and been incorporated within other divisions of DHS. Nevertheless, the purchaser–funder–provider split remains, and the functions of the three units are essentially unchanged.

As previously indicated, probably the most controversial aspect of the restructure was the decision to put area services out to public tender in 1997. As a result, the non-government agencies which had been accustomed to annual grants for their foster care services were forced to compete with one another for one or more of the area services. The further requirement for the successful tenderer to accept all referrals no matter the number added to the antipathy that some of the potential 'providers' already felt towards the restructure. When all of the tenders were reviewed by the Community Services Division, it was decided to award the two metropolitan area services to two different providers. However, after intense lobbying of the then Minister for Family and Community Services by Anglicare SA, the decision of the Tender Board was overturned and both metropolitan areas were awarded to Anglicare. Anglicare SA is the welfare arm of the Church with which the Minister himself was affiliated. Naturally the other non-government agencies viewed the Minister's behaviour as a betrayal of trust, and the bitterness over the way the contract was ultimately won remains within the sector to this day.

The foster care tender was duly let over the vocal objections of Anglicare's competitors in December 1997, and the foster carers who had previously been affiliated with the unsuccessful agencies were transferred to Anglicare.

Summary

In summary, then, the government's retreat from alternative care, which began almost two decades ago, reached its climax in 1997 with the outsourcing of foster care services to the non-government sector. What began primarily as an attempt to reduce government outlays on welfare by transferring out-of-home care from the (mainly government) residential sector to individual foster families has evolved over the years into a radical redefinition of the role of the state. Through the application of the purchaser–provider model, the government successfully created a quasi-market in alternative care in which the state has managed to shed responsibility for a crisis which is largely of its own making. But the demographic data summarized earlier indicate that the state is not the only party withdrawing from care; so too is the community at large. It is an irony of the purchaser–provider model, with all of its talk about markets and commercial contracts, that its application to foster care ultimately relies on non-paid volunteers. And the supply of volunteer carers, which is already critical, will shrink still further as this generation of carers enters old age. As the volunteer labour supply contracts, the state has only a limited range of options before it. It must: (1) provide more support services and higher levels of remuneration to potential carers, (2) reverse the decline in residential care or (3) reduce the number of children accepted into care. As the first two options obviously require a considerable expansion in government outlays on welfare, it is tempting to predict an increase in youth homelessness roughly proportional to the decrease in available carers in the years ahead.

From the government's viewpoint, however, there is a double benefit in the new arrangements. Not only can it now rely on the acquiescence of the non-government sector but it is in a position to blame that same sector for the demise of foster care. As one despairing 'provider' put it soon after the alternative care tender was let, 'They [the Department of Human Services] handed us a wreck and they have been demanding to know why it's broken ever since'. In Chapter 6, we show that, although FAYS workers expressed a great deal of discontent about working in foster care, most also acknowledged that most of the problems were not new.

What has happened to foster care in South Australia also shows that transfer of responsibility via outsourcing does not necessarily mean loss of control; in fact, the opposite is the case in foster care. The combination of service agreements lasting only a few years at a time with tightly prescribed contractual obligations effectively reduces the non-government sector to agents of the state. Either the non-government agencies comply with the edicts of the purchaser or they face financial ruin. If the danger of grants-based funding was that the non-government sector was insufficiently accountable, then the danger of competitive tendering is precisely the opposite – that the non-government sector is utterly beholden to the state. In just one example of this subservience, when policies governing such crucial areas as allegations of abuse in care were being developed, for example, foster care agencies were never consulted despite the fact that they were named as co-investigators in the development process. Moreover, the foster care policy manual that was developed unilaterally by FAYS was not provided to foster care providers until after the system had been implemented. These incidents illustrate that one of the most regrettable casualties of the 'purchaser-provider' approach to foster care has been co-operation – co-operation between government and non-government agencies, and between non-government agencies themselves.

Chapter 4

Methodology

Overview

This chapter summarizes the methodology employed in our tracking study of children in foster care. The first part of the chapter provides a critical overview of the conceptual issues that must be considered when undertaking any kind of evaluation research in the field of alternative care. This first section also describes the analytical framework that was developed for the study as a whole. The second part of the chapter then provides a detailed description of the methodology and the measures on which most of the later chapters are based.

Towards an analytical framework

Welfare services are complex systems, involving the interaction of different individuals, multiple service providers, and different levels of government. With this in mind, it is unwise to expect that the quality of the system as a whole can be understood merely in terms of one area of performance, or that individuals in one part of the system will necessarily be aware of what happens in other areas. For these reasons, an eclectic or mixed methodology approach is required; one that can not only incorporate the various components of the system but also take advantage of the different sources of data that are available through the system.

There are also fundamental decisions to be taken about the precise focus of a study into the outcomes of foster care. Generally speaking, when the term 'outcome' is used within the field of child welfare, it is either too narrowly defined or confused with related terms such as 'output' or 'goal'. In Courtney's view (1993), the outcomes of alternative care should be broken into three separate components: (1) the characteristics of the services provided, (2) the quality of case processes and (3) the case outcomes. Table 4.1 presents these components together with illustrations of performance indicators relevant to each of them. The first component, service characteristics, refers mainly to the quality of placements provided. This includes not only

Table 4.1 Key performance areas in the evaluation of alternative care

Performance area	Indicator variables
Service characteristics	Quality of care environment, staff training and ratio of children to carers
Case processes	Quality of casework, frequency of contact, quality of support and services provided
Case outcomes	
Case status	Legal status, reunified versus in care, type of care, stability of placements
Client outcomes	Psychosocial and educational functioning
Child satisfaction	Child's goals, wishes and needs

the physical and social environment of the placement but also the ratio of children to carers and the qualifications of those providing the care. The second area, case processes, refers to the quality of assistance provided by social workers charged with the task of managing each placement. Performance in this sense refers to the quality of case planning, the frequency with which caseworkers are in contact with children and carers, and the general quality of the relationship between social workers and the children under their care.

The third area, case outcomes, is the primary focus of this book and it can be further divided into three elements (Magura and Moses 1986): case status, client outcomes and child satisfaction. Case status refers to the child's legal or placement status, and includes the type of order that applies, whether the child is still in care or reunified with family and the type of placement arrangement (e.g., foster care versus residential care). The concept of client outcomes refers predominantly to the psychosocial well-being of the child, namely, how the child's general well-being or development has been influenced by the experience of being in care. Because externally administered assessments of well-being do not always coincide with the views of children in care, a final component of outcome evaluation recommended by Courtney (1993) involves administration of child satisfaction measures to determine the extent to which alternative care services have met the client's needs, expectations and wishes.

All of these aspects of outcome evaluation were operationalized in our project through a combination of qualitative and quantitative research methods and through the use of primary and secondary data sources. More specifically, the project involved a focus group study with service providers and carers, semi-structured interviews with foster children and carers, the administration of standardized measures to social workers and carers and interrogation of agency databases and case files.

The focus group study of workers and carers

Overview

The first component of our evaluation involved a series of focus groups with workers and foster carers. Groups were conducted with FAYS workers and foster care agencies in regional and metropolitan South Australia. (South Australia has a population of 1.5 million. The capital, Adelaide, has a population of approximately 1 million.) These forums included participants from most service providers in the alternative care system described in Chapter 3, including FAYS social workers, managers of FAYS District Centres, the Central Alternative Care Unit and representatives from the foster care provider agencies. The focus groups commenced in 1998, and most were held every quarter for twelve months. Separate focus groups were held with workers from different geographical areas, both within the metropolitan area and across the regional areas.

Sampling and procedure for worker groups

Offices of the Department of Family and Youth Services were contacted and invited to participate in focus group discussions. Each office was asked to obtain a sample of volunteer participants from all service areas, and all levels of management. Included in each FAYS group of six to eight was an office supervisor, a senior practitioner, and representatives from each service area in the office: intake and assessment, adolescent workers and child protection. A similar methodology was employed to gauge the views of the foster care agencies. Both support workers and managers were interviewed to enhance the breadth of the views expressed and the issues discussed. These selection procedures accord with common recommendations concerning the conduct of qualitative interviews involving organizations (Shadbolt and Burton 1990). The inclusion of managers in the focus group, for example, provided insight into the general operation of the system, including the extent to which broader policy imperatives were being implemented at an office level. Practitioners, on the other hand, were included to obtain details about day-to-day problem-solving, and, in particular, examples of practice issues and cases illustrating the difficulties of the new foster care system.

　Each focus group lasted between one and two hours and was chaired by a moderator from the research project. Sessions consisted of a brief introduction followed by a semi-directed discussion of broad questions relating to changes in service delivery and worker roles since the introduction of the new system. These questions were not asked in any particular order, but were introduced according to the general flow and context of the discussion. For each general question, there was a list of specific points that the moderator could use as prompts to guide and stimulate discussion. A summary of the general questions is provided in Table 4.2.

Table 4.2 Questions used in worker focus groups

FAYS workers

1	How would you describe the tasks of the district centre worker as the allocated worker in alternative care? Has this changed with the restructuring of alternative care?
2	Has your direct work with children in care, birth families and foster families changed with restructuring of alternative care? How has it changed? Have you got any cases which exemplify the issues you are raising?
3	Has the service delivery changed and what are some of the changes you have noted?
4	What is the personal impact of restructuring on you?
5	With the benefit of hindsight, would you have done anything differently?

Foster care workers

1	How would you describe the tasks of the allocated case worker as the allocated worker in alternative care? Have these changed with the restructuring of alternative care?
2	Has your direct work with children in care, birth families and foster families changed with restructuring of alternative care? How has it changed? Have you got any cases which exemplify the issues you are raising?
3	If you were working in alternative care before the restructuring, how has your work changed?
4	What is the personal impact of restructuring on you?
5	With the benefit of hindsight would you have done anything different?

Each focus group was audiotaped and the discussions were transcribed in full. Key themes were then identified by project staff and the authors compiled a full list of points relating to each theme to determine which issues were raised most often, and by which agency. A summary of the resultant themes is presented in Chapter 5.

Sampling and procedure for carer groups

Two carer focus groups were conducted with a purposive sample of carers within the first twelve months of the restructure of foster care described in Chapter 3. The names of approximately thirty-five foster carers were taken from the list of carers attached to South Australia's largest foster care agency, Anglicare SA. Carers were chosen by the research team to provide a mix of rural and metropolitan carers, as well as carers who were either new to fostering or who had provided care both before and after the restructure. Finally, the names chosen also represented a mix of carers to 'protected' and 'disaffected' children (see Chapter 5). Carers were invited to attend a focus group discussion of their experiences and were provided with two

Table 4.3 Questions used in carer focus groups

1	For those of you who provided foster care under the old system, what are some of the differences between the old and the new system?
2	Are there any comments about recruitment and training in the new system?
3	What support do you get under the new system?
4	Do you feel valued as a foster carer?
5	Do you have any comments about how decisions are made regarding the child in your care?
6	With the benefit of hindsight, what, if anything, should Anglicare and FAYS have done differently with this new system?

possible times to attend. Unfortunately, the first of these times clashed with another function that was being held by the agency and attendance at this group was very small ($n = 5$) but the second group was attended by 20 carers. Carer focus groups also lasted between one and two hours and were chaired by a moderator from the research project. Sessions again consisted of a brief introduction followed by a discussion of broad questions that were introduced in a different order on both occasions. A summary of these discussion questions is provided in Table 4.3.

The tracking study of children in care

Introduction

The purpose of the second and major part of the project was to obtain detailed information concerning the placement movements and psychosocial outcomes of children in foster care. Although studies of this kind have been conducted before, a limitation of most of them has been their reliance on cross-sectional designs (see Altshuler and Gleeson 1999 for a review). Most often, the functioning of children in care has been compared with that of children in the general population or comparable groups in the child welfare system at a single point in time (Kinard 1994). Such designs provide no adequate baseline against which to compare change and often lead to sampling bias by over-representing children with longer and more unstable placement histories (Courtney 1994; Goerge 1990). This is problematic because children with long placement histories often have other characteristics that distinguish them from the rest of the children in care. For example, long-stay children tend to be older and often display poorer levels of psychosocial adjustment than short-stay children. Thus, cross-sectional analyses involving 'snapshot' profiles of children in care may provide an overly pessimistic view of long-term experiences and outcomes. This issue has led researchers to advocate longitudinal designs that allow for comparison of outcomes over time. Most of the longitudinal studies that have been conducted to date, however, have been retrospective. Data have usually been obtained from large archival datasets, such as those routinely maintained by agencies, and used to generate social indicators of various kinds (Courtney 1994, 1995a; Courtney and Wong 1996; Fernandez 1999; Goerge 1990). Although these studies have proved highly effective in predicting changes in case status over time, they have been limited by the range of variables included, the sophistication of the measures available and the absence of follow-up measures more proximal to the outcomes predicted. For example, it is questionable whether particular outcomes can be confidently associated with factors such as abuse that may have occurred years earlier.

In contrast, prospective longitudinal designs not only make possible comparisons with a consistent baseline but they are also in a position to collect a greater volume of information and to choose the information that is collected. Although concerns can be raised about potential biases resulting from the selective loss of subjects over time, a prospective study has the capacity to identify, and potentially control for, any systematic differences between the retained sample and those who drop out. Testament to the effectiveness of the prospective longitudinal design is the oft-cited study undertaken by Fanshel and Shinn (1978), who tracked the progress of over six hundred New York children placed into care during the late 1960s. In that study, outcome measures were administered annually for a total of five years, thereby making it possible to assess changes in psychosocial adjustment and placement outcomes across time.

Despite the fact that child welfare legislation everywhere advances child well-being as its most fundamental objective, efforts to measure the well-being of children in state care have been surprisingly rare and unsustained. Altshuler and Gleeson (1999), for example, recently noted that measures of success in foster care have been dominated by indicators of permanency and safety, while child well-being is rarely incorporated into administrative databases or built into the evaluation of system performance. No doubt one of the reasons for this omission is that, whereas permanency and safety can be safely inferred from administrative data such as abuse and re-referral rates, the measurement of child well-being is more subjective and potentially more labour-intensive (Courtney 1993; Magura and Moses 1986). In other words, and in terms of the framework described earlier, there is considerably more information available concerning changes in case status than there is about variations in client outcomes. Analysis of case status information is useful because it provides one indicator of how the system is operating in relation to broader policy objectives. Assuming that placement stability and family reunification are global policy objectives, it can be useful to know how many, or how soon, children return home, and how many placement changes occur along the way. However, it is crucial that these objectives do not become ends in themselves. Although it is reasonable to suggest that early reunificiation and placement stability should, *ceteris paribus*, lead to better psychosocial outcomes, it does not necessarily follow that this will be so. To illustrate the point, Courtney (1993) drew attention to New York City's Program Assessment System implemented in the early 1980s, in which agency performance was linked solely to statistical criteria such as the number of children in alternative care and the speed of their reunification. This system led to a situation in which the quality of care was compromised in the interests of maintaining a criterion rate of reunification. Children were sent home early wherever possible, often without due regard to their safety, and agencies were reluctant to accept difficult children because such children were less likely to be reunified and this, in turn, would reduce the agency's putative performance and funding entitlements.

In response to the limitations of case status data, Courtney (1993), Barber and Delfabbro (2000a) and Zill and Coiro (1992) have all argued that there is a need for more direct, standardized measures of child well-being in care. In order to achieve this objective, several important issues need to be considered. The first of these is the comprehensiveness of the assessment, and the second is the efficiency or practicality of the measures. By comprehensiveness, we are referring to the objective that assessments should not be confined to any single measure but should encompass all of the critical domains of psychosocial development encapsulated within the concept of well-being. This includes not only physical and psychological health but also social functioning, education and behavioural adjustment. Zill and Coiro (1992) provide a number of examples of how these variables might be captured, including:

- assessments of physical health status based upon the frequency of check-ups and general health ratings
- educational performance assessed by estimates of school attendance, grades and IQ tests
- social adjustment measured by ratings of the effectiveness of the child's interactions with others, e.g. the child's co-operativeness, popularity and responsiveness towards others
- emotional adjustment assessed using measures such as Achenbach's (1991) Child Behavior Checklist (CBCL) with a particular focus on antisocial and destructive behaviours, emotionality and hyperactivity.

As Barber and Delfabbro (2000a) and McDonald et al. (1996) point out, however, the difficulty with these recommendations, particularly in relation to measures of emotional well-being, is that most of the commonly advocated measures such as the Child Well-Being Scales (Magura and Moses 1986) and the CBCL are too laborious to be used for routine assessment. There is a need for briefer, more usable measures to be developed, measures that can be incorporated into the day-to-day casework of child welfare professionals. This chapter reports on the development of abbreviated CBCL sub-scales which meet this criterion. Boyle and Jones (1985) have also argued that there is frequently a lack of connection between the applications of child well-being measures and the context in which they were originally developed. A measure such as the CBCL, for example, was developed predominantly for use in clinical settings, so it is unclear whether the items are necessarily representative of the types of behaviour commonly observed in alternative care settings.

A further consideration relates to the difficulty associated with conducting the assessment itself, particularly identifying the most reliable source from which child well-being data can be collected. Although detailed case file information is frequently available in child welfare agencies, this information is more often than not inconsistently recorded, inaccurate or incomplete. There is also no systematic way in which this information can be compiled and standardized so that useful comparisons can be made across children (Magura and Moses 1986). Accordingly, it is necessary to obtain data from people who have close contact with the child. The three most obvious choices in this regard are social workers, foster carers and children themselves. None of these sources is entirely without problems, of course. Foster carers, for example, are normally highly motivated to improve the life circumstances of the children in their care and this can show up as a bias towards improved well-being scores over time. As external observers, social workers might be capable of more objective judgements but they do not live with the child, so their knowledge of the child's progress may not be sufficiently detailed for valid assessments to be made. Finally, children may be reluctant to put their placements in a negative light for fear that any such information could be used against them, or passed on to their carers. For these reasons, both Courtney (1993) and Zill and Coiro (1992) advocate the accumulation of information from multiple sources.

Our approach to the study was guided by the methodological issues considered above. Most importantly, a longitudinal cohort study was chosen in recognition of the potential biases associated with cross-sectional designs. In addition, the study included baseline and follow-up measures of all client outcome measures recommended in Table 4.1.

Sample selection

The tracking study involved 235 children (121 boys, 114 girls) with a mean age of 10.8 years and an age range of four to seventeen years. Children were selected if they were referred for a new placement between May 1998 and April 1999. Excluded from the sample were children on detention orders, children in supported accommodation, those referred for family preservation services and those with placements of less than two weeks' duration. The exclusion of very young children is consistent with the recommendations of Zill and Coiro (1992), who argue that psychosocial assessment is very difficult with pre-school children, and that measures that are valid for the four to seventeen age group are not valid for infants. The final sample represented the entire cohort of children meeting the selection criteria referred via the central referral agency (see Chapter 3) for both metropolitan and regional areas of South Australia. The sample consisted of 40 (17 per cent) Aboriginal children and 195 (83 per cent) non-Aboriginal children. Sixty-three (27 per cent) were from the country areas of South Australia and 171 (73 per cent) were from the metropolitan area of Adelaide. A breakdown of the sample by age showed that 65 (27.5 per cent) were aged from four to eight years, 79 (33.7 per cent) were aged nine to twelve years and 90 (37.6 per cent) were aged thirteen to seventeen years. Of the children, 37 per cent ($n = 86$) were referred on short-term legal orders (up to twelve months), and the rest, 149 (63 per cent), were on longer-term orders of at least twelve months' duration.

Referral records at the Central Alternative Care Unit (CACU) were monitored each week. The data for children selected for inclusion were recorded together with the contact details and location of the FAYS workers responsible for each case. This information was collected from central agency records and government databases and was verified with FAYS workers in interviews. FAYS workers were contacted within two weeks of the initial referral and face-to-face interviews were arranged at the local offices. In those few cases that involved delayed placement, the interview was postponed until such time as the central payment records indicated that a placement had commenced.

After the intake interview, follow-up interviews were conducted with FAYS workers (Figure 4.1). The first of these follow-ups occurred four months after the intake interview. A second interview occurred at eight months, a third at twelve months, and then interviews were undertaken every six months thereafter. Given that the full cohort was not collected until May 1999, children who came into the study last were tracked for only two years, compared with three years for those who had entered at the start of the sampling period (May 1998). For this reason, the analyses described in later chapters are largely confined to a two-year period in the interests of consistency and sample size. Cases were tracked as long as they remained 'open' from the point of view of the South Australian Department of Family and Youth Services. Children therefore remained in the study irrespective of

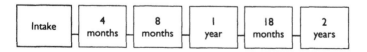

Figure 4.1 Follow-up points in the tracking study

their placement status, as long as there was an allocated worker from whom information could be obtained. Tracking ceased only when children had returned home or been discharged, the case had been closed for at least one month and there was also no longer a worker available with recent knowledge of the case.

Data collection at intake

Most of the information captured in intake assessments was collected either from case files or in the course of the interviews lasting one to two hours that were routinely conducted with the FAYS worker responsible for referring the child into care. The variables covered by intake assessments included the following: demographic characteristics; client status variables; placement history; significant problems; family contact plan; degree of dislocation; cognitive functioning; education; offending behaviour (children aged ten years or older only); general physical health; substance abuse; sexualized behaviours; conduct disorder scale; hyperactivity scale; emotionality scale; social adjustment; and education.

Demographic characteristics. These items were extracted from case files and included the child's gender, age and ethnicity; and whether the child had been referred from a metropolitan or regional area.

Client status variables. These variables included: the nature of the legal order that applied (for example, 'voluntary custody', 'parental authority' agreements not involving a court order or court-ordered 'guardianships' of twelve months or longer) and the nature of the initial placement (for example, foster care, relative care or residential care).

Placement history. On the basis of central computer records, it was possible to ascertain the approximate number of placements children had experienced previously, as well as how long (in months) they had been in care. This allowed children to be classified into one of three groups: 'new into care', 'returning to care' or 'changing placement' (referred for a new placement as a result of a placement breakdown).

Significant problems. A variety of problems pertaining to the child and the circumstances of the placement were identified by social workers at intake. The first of these related to whether children had been victims of any form of abuse, physical, sexual, emotional, and/or neglect. *Child incapacity* was used to describe cases in which children had significant physical or mental health problems; *child mental health* referred to cases in which children were experiencing severe depression, suicidal ideation or self-harming behaviours; *parental incapacity* referred to cases in which parents were in prison, had substance abuse problems or had mental or physical illness; *family breakdown* referred to cases involving severe child–parent conflict; and finally, *child behaviour* referred to cases of children with problematic behaviours at the time of the reference placement.

Family contact plan.   FAYS workers were also asked to indicate the frequency of planned contact between the child and his or her birth family during the placement. Three types of contact were distinguished: telephone or letters (indirect), visits (direct) and overnight stays. For each of these, contact frequency was recorded on a five-point scale where 1 = never, 2 = monthly or less often, 3 = 2–3 times a month, 4 = once a week, 5 = 2–6 times a week, and 7 = daily.

Degree of dislocation.   FAYS workers were asked to indicate whether the child did or did not need to change school as a result of the referral, and how far the placement was from the child's birth family: 1 = < 5 km, 2 = 5–10 km, 3 = 11–20 km, 4 = 21–50 km, 5 = 51+ km.

Cognitive functioning.   FAYS workers were asked whether the child's cognitive abilities had been formally assessed by a psychologist. IQ scores were recorded wherever this information was available. The information was not available for many children, and assessments were generally not undertaken for any children in care for less than twelve months.

Education.   Respondents were also asked whether the children were in education and, if so, the type of education (pre-school, primary, high-school or other) and the grade-level. They were also asked to rate the child's recent academic performance compared with his or her peers on a seven-point scale (1 = bottom of the class, 4 = average, 7 = top of the class). If the child was not attending school, workers were asked to indicate why this was so on a short checklist which included: left school, excluded, school refusal. Finally, workers were asked to indicate how many times the child had changed school, been suspended or excluded during the twelve months prior to entering the study.

Offending behaviour (children aged ten years or older only).   The interview schedule asked FAYS workers to indicate how often the children had been convicted of an offence in the twelve months prior to the study. They were then asked to indicate (on a checklist) the type of offence that had been committed. This checklist included: theft, damaging property, sexual and physical assault, disorderly conduct, arson, car offences and an open category for other types of offence. Because offending behaviour occurred so rarely in our sample, there was little point in including these data in the analyses reported in this book.

General physical health.   The child's overall level of physical health during the previous three months was assessed on a four-point scale where 1 = healthy all of the time, 2 = healthy most of the time, 3 = healthy only some of the time, and 4 = not at all healthy. If a rating of 3 or 4 was reported, FAYS workers were provided with a checklist and asked to indicate which symptoms had been experienced by the child, and how often. As with offending behaviour, the rate of sickness in our sample was so low that this variable was also excluded from data analysis.

Substance abuse.   The frequency with which children and adolescents were drinking alcohol without adult supervision, using marijuana or other drugs, sniffing glue or solvents, or misusing prescription medications was also recorded. A four-item scale was used for each substance, where 1 = never, 2 = once a month or less often, 3 = 2–3 times a month, 4 = weekly or more often. This yielded a scale that ranged from 4 (no substance use) to 16 (frequent substance use). The scale alpha for this scale was > 0.80 at all assessment points. Little could be done with this variable because substance use was so rarely reported within our sample.

Sexualized behaviours.   FAYS workers were also asked to indicate whether children were putting themselves at risk or engaging in inappropriate sexualized behaviours. Items included: inappropriate sexualized behaviours (e.g. towards young children or excessive promiscuity towards care givers and other adults), perpetrating sexual abuse, involvement in prostitution or associating with paedophiles. For each of these items, respondents were asked to indicate (yes or no) whether the behaviour had occurred in the previous four months. The scale alpha was > 0.80 at all measurement points.

Conduct disorder scale.   An abbreviated conduct scale was constructed based upon six items drawn from Boyle *et al.*'s (1987) Child Behavior Checklist. These items satisfied the key criteria of the DSM classification for conduct disorder, and each was scored (0 = never, 1 = sometimes, 2 = often) giving a possible total score ranging from 0 to 12 which was divided by the total number of items (six) to yield a mean conduct score of between 0 and 2. The six conduct items referred to: destroying property, damaging property, defiance at school, lying and cheating, stealing from outside the home and physical assault. The scale alpha for this measure was found to be > 0.80 at intake and at every follow-up point thereafter.

Hyperactivity scale.   An abbreviated hyperactivity scale was constructed based upon three items from Boyle *et al.*'s (1987) CBC. These items captured the key elements of the DSM classification for hyperactivity disorder, and each was scored in the same way as the conduct disorder scale (0 = never, 1 = sometimes, 2 = often). The three items were: 'could not concentrate or pay attention for long', 'couldn't sit still, was restless and hyperactive', 'distractible, had trouble sticking to things'. Again, the scale alpha was > 0.80 at all measurement points.

Emotionality scale.   An emotionality scale was constructed which consisted of five items drawn from Boyle *et al.*'s (1987) CBC. These items captured the key elements of the DSM categories relating to 'overanxious disorder' and 'affective disorder'. Each of the five items was scored (0 = never, 1 = sometimes, 2 = often) giving a possible total score of between 0 and 10 which was again divided by the number of items to yield a mean emotionality score between 0 and 2. The items included: 'unhappy, sad or depressed', 'not as happy as other children', 'nervous, highly strung or tense', 'too fearful or anxious' and 'worried a lot'. The scale alpha for this scale was again acceptable (> 0.79) across all measurement points.

The items selected from Boyle *et al.*'s (1987) Child Behavior Checklist to measure conduct disorder, hyperactivity and emotionality were those found by Barber, Bolitho and Bertrand (1999a, b) to have the highest item-total correlations with their relevant sub-scales in a study of over two thousand Canadian adolescents.

Social adjustment.   Social workers were asked to complete a seven-item social adjustment scale previously developed by Barber and Delfabbro (2000b) in a national study of parenting behaviour. The scale consisted of four items relating to social relationships ('Has been getting along with people', 'Has resented people telling him/her what to do', 'Has felt persecuted or picked on', 'Has blamed others for his/her mistakes'), and three items measuring social confidence ('Felt self-confident', 'Has looked forward to mixing with others', 'Has been willing to talk and express feelings'). Each item was scored on a four-point scale (1 = often, 2 = sometimes, 3 = rarely, 4 = never). Items were recoded so that higher scores on all items represented a better level of social adjustment. This generated a scale with a possible total of between 7 (low adjustment) and 28 (high adjustment), which was divided by 7 to produce a mean social adjustment score of between 1 and 4. In Barber and Delfabbro's (2000b) national study, this scale was administered to a stratified random sample of 377 parents and their children. In that study, the scale was found to be internally consistent for both children (alpha = 0.74) and parents (alpha = 0.70). A similar level of internal consistency was found in the present study with social worker reports (alpha > 0.70 at all measurement points).

Education.   Social workers were then administered ten items concerning the child's general educational performance during the previous four months. All items were scored on four-point scales: 1 = often, 2 = sometimes, 3 = rarely, 4 = never. Four items referred to general school performance: 'Has been well-organized', 'Has been interested in his/her studies', 'Has produced work of a good standard', 'Has been attentive in class'. Six items referred to the child's behaviour and level of co-operation: 'Has not completed homework or set work', 'Has been disruptive in class', 'Has refused to take part in school activities', 'Has been disciplined by teachers and other staff members', 'Has been late to class' and 'Has wagged school'. All three of these sub-scales were found to possess acceptable alphas (> 0.70) across all measurement points, although the final items were not combined in a scale format because of the small number of items involved.

Follow-up data collection

At each follow-up point, the foster child's social worker was interviewed again concerning the child's progress in care and all of the scales described above were re-administered. In addition, there were questions that updated the child's placement status ('in same placement', 'changed placement but still in care', 'reunified with family', and other relevant categories, such as 'moved into independent living', 'missing', 'in custody', and so forth). There were also questions that updated the child's legal status, health status, education status (for example, whether the child had changed school or left school, number of school suspensions or exclusions); and questions recording the nature and frequency of offending behaviour.

Family contacts. In relation to birth family interactions, social workers were asked to provide details of the frequency of each type of contact that had occurred since intake (or the previous follow-up point). There were also some questions concerning changes in family relationship and the effects of this contact. Specifically, social workers were asked whether the frequency of contact between the child and his or her birth family had changed (1 = increased, 2 = decreased, 3 = no change), and whether the contacts were beneficial (1 = not beneficial, 2 = somewhat beneficial, 3 = very beneficial). Social workers were also asked about the quality of the relationship between child and birth family since the previous interview (1 = very much improved, 2 = slightly improved, 3 = unchanged, 4 = slightly deteriorated, 5 = very much deteriorated), and about change in the likelihood of reunification since that interview (1 = increased, 2 = decreased, 3 = no change).

Details of placement changes. The most critical addition to follow-up surveys was the inclusion of a substantial section detailing the nature of all placement movements or changes of status. The child's every movement since intake or the previous follow-up (except for respite from an ongoing placement) was recorded and described. This record included the duration of the placement and the circumstances of the change (for example, 'child missing', 'in custody'), the reasons for any changes and the geographical location of each new placement.

Inter-rater reliability of measures

An inter-rater reliability study was conducted during the first year of the project to investigate the accuracy of social worker reports. This involved conducting identical interviews with foster carers as proximal to the social worker interview as possible. One potential criticism of this comparison is that social worker and carer reports represent genuinely different perspectives on the child, and therefore that an exact coincidence of views or ratings should not be expected, particularly when subjective interpretations of the child's emotional state are required. As Courtney (1993) points out, foster carers may be inclined to underestimate the children's emotional problems because they naturally want to portray their homes as friendly and happy places to live. Notwithstanding the potential limitations of an inter-rater reliability study, however, we proceeded with the analysis in the knowledge that items relating to internal states represented only a small proportion of the total items assessed, and that most items referred to objective and highly visible behaviours. In all, carer interviews were completed for 61 children (33 boys and 28 girls) randomly selected from the tracking study. Of the carers selected, only those who had been looking after the child for at least one month were included in the trial. There was good evidence that the majority of both comparison groups were familiar with the cases: there was no significant difference between the amount of time (in months) that social workers had managed the children's cases ($M = 4.98$, $SD = 2.13$) and the amount of time that the children had been living with their foster carers ($M = 5.05$, $SD = 2.25$), $t (60) < 1$. Approximately 90 per cent ($n = 50$) of the social workers and 90 per cent of the foster carers had managed the child's affairs for the full follow-up period (four months) to which the measures applied. Seventy-four per cent ($n = 42$) of social workers were in telephone contact with foster carers at least on a weekly basis, seventeen (28 per cent) were in contact at least once a month, and only three (5 per cent) were in contact less often than once a month. Direct contact between the child and social worker was generally infrequent: 16.7 per cent had direct contact at least on a weekly basis, approximately two-thirds (63 per cent) had contact every two to four weeks, and the remaining 20 per cent had contact less than once a month.

Physical health. On the four-point scale used to measure physical health, a score of 1 or 2 indicated good health (1 = all the time, 2 = most of the time) whereas scores of 3 and 4 indicated poor health (3 = healthy only some of the time, 4 = not at all healthy). Thus, children could be classified into two groups (1 = 'generally healthy' based upon a score of 1 or 2, or 2 = 'generally unhealthy', based upon a score of 3 or 4). Of a total of 60 valid comparions, 56 (93 per cent) of the children were classified as generally healthy by both sources, and 2 (3 per cent) were classified by both as generally unhealthy. Thus, 96 per cent of the health classifications were identical.

Substance use. As previously discussed, the use of psychoactive substances was measured on four-point scales: 1 = never, 2 = less than monthly, 3 = 2–3 times a month, 4 = weekly or more often. Owing to the limited opportunity for substance abuse during foster care placements, very few of these behaviours were observed. Thus, children were classified as frequent (2–3 times per month or more often) or infrequent users (once per month or less often) for each of the four substances. A comparison of the frequencies in each group revealed a very high level of agreement between the carers and social workers (mean percentage agreement = 96 per cent).

Sexualized behaviours. Once again, there was very high correspondence between the two sources with very little evidence of under-reporting or over-reporting by social workers relative to carers. The mean overall level of agreement was 97 per cent.

Psychological adjustment (conduct disorder, hyperactivity and emotionality). Items on each of these scales were scored on a three-point scale with 1 = never, 2 = sometimes, 3 = often. Consistent with the above analyses, children were classified into two groups: those where both sources agreed that the behaviour had not occurred (scores of 1), and those where both agreed that the behaviour had occurred (scores of 2 and 3). The results showed that over 70 per cent of responses for conduct disorder and hyperactivity corresponded exactly, although social workers somewhat under-reported issues of conduct disorder relative to carers. This difference, averaged across all items, was approximately 9 per cent, meaning that just over one in ten ratings made by social workers would be considered by carers to be false negatives (the omission of behavioural events reported by foster carers). The overall correspondence for emotionality items was somewhat weaker. Although both sources agreed about the presence or absence of items measuring depression (78 per cent agreement), the percentage agreement for other items (for example, 'child worries a lot') was no better than chance. An encouraging observation, however, was that these differences were in a consistent direction: for all items, poor emotional functioning was significantly more likely to be reported by social workers than by foster carers.

Social adjustment. Each social adjustment item was rated on a four-point scale: 1 = often, 2 = sometimes, 3 = rarely, 4 = never. Once again, children were classified into two groups: those where both sources agreed that the behaviour had occurred at least sometimes (score of 1 or 2), and those where both sources believed that the behaviour had rarely or never occurred (scores of 3 or 4). The level of agreement between the two sources varied significantly across items. Approximately 90 per cent of foster carers and social workers agreed on items measuring visible aspects of social functioning ('gets along well with people', 'looks forward to mixing with others').

They also generally agreed about items relating to the child's general disposition towards others ('resents being told what to do'). Once again, however, the level of correspondence was less satisfactory (approximately 60 per cent) for items relating to internalized behaviours ('blames others for mistakes', 'is willing to express feelings').

Educational adjustment. Each educational adjustment item was scored in the same way as the social adjustment items and, in general, there was satisfactory correspondence between the two sets of ratings. Over 70 per cent of foster carers and social workers agreed that each behaviour had, or had not, occurred. The only exception was for items relating to more specific behaviours such as 'not taking part in activities', where the degree of correspondence fell to only 56 per cent.

Taken as a whole, then, the results of the reliability evaluation were encouraging. For items relating to factual or highly visible behaviours, there was a satisfactory level of agreement between social worker and foster carer reports. Furthermore, in domains where the level of agreement was poorer, the nature of the difference was generally in the expected direction and probably reflects genuine differences in the experiences of the two groups rather than deficiencies in social workers' knowledge of the child.

The consumer feedback studies

Embedded within the larger tracking study were two smaller consumer feedback studies. In the first of these, 51 children in short- to medium-term care (23 girls, 28 boys) were interviewed using a semi-structured format to assess their satisfaction with their placements. Twelve of the children were in residential care at the time of interview and 39 were in foster placements. These children were selected, on the basis of FAYS' approval and availability, from our longitudinal study cohort. The children were interviewed approximately six months after they entered the study and were asked a number of questions relating to their satisfaction with their social worker, such as whether or not they knew the name of their FAYS worker, how often they saw that worker, whether their worker listened to them and cared for them, and how helpful their worker had been. Children were also asked to rate their current placement on various dimensions, including security satisfaction and care giving received.

In the second study, a total of 48 children (23 girls, 25 boys) in long-term care were interviewed. These children were again selected from the larger tracking study on the basis of availability and capacity to answer questions about their well-being. In this study, the children's social workers were administered the conduct disorder scale described above and the children were administered a standardized measure of child satisfaction derived from Stuntzner-Gibson, Koren and DeChillo (1995). This latter measure consists of eleven items relating to the child's satisfaction with placement, including whether the child liked living with the foster family, was able to get help and have fun, and felt supported.

Further methodological details on both consumer feedback studies are provided in Chapter 7, where the results are presented.

Interviews with disruptive children and their carers

In the course of our tracking study, we became aware of a group of children who had been very poorly served by foster care. Most of these children were adolescents who had entered the foster care system with some level of conduct disorder and/or disability (see Chapter 10). In an effort to find out more than the statistical data could tell us about these children, we conducted in-depth interviews with 13 of them. The children were aged between ten and seventeen years and had experienced at least one shortened placement, ostensibly because the carer had found the child's behaviour intolerable. Interviews with the children covered: (1) the circumstances leading up to placement breakdown, (2) the point at which placement problems first became apparent to the child, (3) the child's emotional response to the breakdown, (4) whether and with whom the child had discussed placement problems, (5) positive and negative aspects of the placement, and (6) whether, in the child's view, any intervention might have enabled the placement to continue. Similar questions were put to nineteen carers who had terminated placements because of the child's behaviour and the responses were compared. The findings of this study, together with the relevant methodological details, are presented in Chapter 11.

Part III

Results

Chapter 5

The views of workers and carers on outsourced care

Introduction

Ever since South Australian foster care was outsourced in 1997 (see Chapter 3), there has been a strict division of responsibility between the statutory agency, Family and Youth Service (FAYS), that requests placements for its children and the non-government providers of that care. Under the new system, FAYS workers who require a foster placement must now refer the child to the Central Alternative Care Unit (CACU), which processes the referral information without ever actually meeting the child and then contacts one or other of the foster care agencies to negotiate a suitable placement. CACU is an autonomous unit within FAYS, whose role is to exercise some degree of quality control over the information provided to foster care agencies and, through them, to carers. CACU also aims to promote equity in the system by preventing FAYS workers from competing with one another for placements. In fact, verbal communication between FAYS workers and foster care agencies is proscribed until after CACU has secured a placement. The only way that FAYS workers are supposed to convey the placement needs of children to the foster care agencies is by way of a referral form which is provided to CACU.

In this chapter, we report on the experiences of foster care workers and carers under the restructured system as those experiences were communicated to us in the focus group discussions outlined in the previous chapter.

The views of workers

The workers responsible for administering South Australia's foster care system complained of many problems with the new arrangements, but underlying most of them was the workers' discomfort with the division between the 'purchasers' and 'providers' of foster care. Workers also complained of communication problems under the new system and of an overemphasis on paperwork at the expense of case planning and social work practice. Another theme to emerge in our discussions with workers, particularly within

FAYS' groups, concerned an alleged decline in the quality of foster placements following outsourcing. Finally, some of the focus groups discussed the very common perception that outsourcing itself had been a ploy by the state to pass responsibility for the parlous state of alternative care to the non-government sector. In the sections that follow, we deal briefly with each of these key themes.

The demarcation of roles

Arguably the most fundamental feature of South Australia's new foster care system is the division of labour between FAYS social workers and foster care workers or, as the latter are more commonly called, Placement Support Workers (PSWs). Under the new arrangements, FAYS workers are responsible for all decisions affecting the welfare of the child, while PSWs are responsible for the support of carers. Theoretically, then, any problem or issue affecting the child should be handled by the FAYS worker, and only by the FAYS worker, while any problem or issue affecting the carer should be handled by the PSW. Even a moment's reflection should be sufficient to convince anyone who has ever actually lived in a family, however, that this is not how families work: a problem for the child is also a problem for the parent and vice versa. Moreover, very many of the problems that arise in families concern *interactions* between parents and children. So whose problem is that? Certainly the FAYS Manual of Practice advises, even insists, that both parties should work together towards the resolution of problems that arise in placement, but this same document also enshrines the division of labour between FAYS workers and PSWs (Family and Youth Services 1997). At best, then, the message is a mixed one.

FAYS staff told us that they were aware of the principle that their responsibility should be to the child, and foster care agencies to the carers, but both FAYS workers and PSWs found the demarcation near impossible to effect in practice. As one FAYS worker put it, 'roles and responsibilities . . . [have to be] negotiated around each individual child and with each individual worker. There is no consistency.' Some FAYS workers felt that their Department had become much too narrow in its focus and needed to take more responsibility for carers, while others held the opposite view. Interestingly, FAYS workers even expressed confusion about new role demarcations within their own Department. Given the very high turnover of placements (see Chapter 7), it was common for foster children to move repeatedly from one FAYS region to another. In some of these situations, the original worker kept the case and dealt with it from across town, while in other cases the child's management was transferred to the new District Centres. In the latter case, workers in the second office often complained that not all of the necessary information about the child was being transferred.

A number of FAYS workers described the new system as 'crisis-driven', implying that most of their work involved responding to emergencies such as placement breakdown rather than providing a social work service. Most of these workers attributed the problem not only to a lack of time for case planning but also to the difficulties associated with trying to work collaboratively with all of the parties involved: no longer just children, birth families and foster carers but also now PSWs and CACU staff as well. In particular, FAYS workers expressed frustration at calling case planning meetings and case conferences only to find that almost none of the relevant parties would turn up. There was a pervasive view that until there was greater continuity in the relationship between FAYS workers and PSWs in particular, the system would continue to be dysfunctional.

Indirect and inadequate communication

Many of us who studied undergraduate psychology were introduced to social psychology with a game of 'Chinese Whispers' in which one person is given a message and asked to convey it secretly to the next person who conveys it in turn to the next person and so on until everyone in the group has had a chance to pass on the message. When the last person in the chain is asked to tell the whole group what they have just been told, there is normally great amusement when the final message is found to bear only a faint resemblance to the original one. This well-worn experiment was invoked more than once by our focus group participants to convey what they believed had happened to communication since the restructure. FAYS workers believed that their knowledge of carers and placements had significantly decreased and that information passed to CACU was being either lost or not conveyed to the foster care agencies. Foster care workers (both managers and PSWs) felt that the old informal system of contact where FAYS workers and PSWs negotiated directly with each other had been much more conducive to quality placements. FAYS and foster care workers were generally in agreement that CACU was partly to blame for the strained relations in the sector, and, although most focus groups were sympathetic to individual CACU staff, most were opposed to the unit in principle. In essence, CACU was seen as a redundant and needlessly bureaucratic obstacle in the referral process. It led to double-handling of information, added an additional level of complexity, contributed to miscommunication and fuelled misunderstanding. Through no fault of their own, CACU staff were said to be insufficiently familiar with the child when making referrals. As a result, it was alleged that absurd placements were sometimes being arranged and foster carers often knew very little about the children who turned up on their doorsteps. Chapter 11 provides alarming, albeit anecdotal, evidence of this phenomenon, such as the case of a foster carer whose sister had been immolated in a house fire but the carer had never been told that the boy she had been assigned was in the habit of setting fires when he was upset. The boy duly did set fire to his carer's house (as FAYS workers suspected he might do) and the carer was so traumatized by the incident that she withdrew from the foster care system.

At the time of our interviews, both FAYS and contracted agencies were actively undermining the work of CACU by developing strategies to circumvent the unit altogether. FAYS and foster care workers argued that it was much easier to speak directly with each other, rather than go via CACU. They blamed CACU for unnecessary delays in the placement process and expressed doubts about CACU's contribution either to equity or to placement quality. CACU countered that they were repeatedly forced to make placements with insufficient referral information from FAYS workers who neglected to complete the necessary referral forms. Even when written information was provided, CACU staff alleged that different offices had their own ways of recording the information and were generally unreceptive to the idea of standardizing the information recorded.

Generally speaking, then, one major casualty of the restructure seems to have been information, which most workers agreed had been seriously eroded under the new arrangements. As one frustrated CACU worker put it:

> You start a referral and if the referral is very sloppy, then you spend all your time ringing that [FAYS] person to find out more information and then you fax it to the [foster care agency]. You ask them both to ring you back and they don't ring you back; there is always an answering machine ... I mean, this morning I had a referral for five children to be placed through the week and it was very clearly on the form that we want to know the reason for it. Yet there was no reason and no signature. I rang the [FAYS] worker; the worker wasn't there; the supervisor wasn't there. All that takes a lot of time. Imagine if five or six referrals come in at once!

As this quotation also shows, even the information that was provided to CACU had to be transferred in hard copy form via fax machine, with workers going through all of the documentation provided by FAYS workers and coding some of it into electronic form for their own purposes. The process was a very protracted one and arguments soon arose between workers about whether or not foster care agencies should be allowed access to all of the available information. In the early stages, FAYS imposed a rigid set of guidelines governing access to and transfer of information between agencies but eventually designed a more flexible system when the former proved unworkable.

Pen-pushing and paper-shuffling

FAYS workers and PSWs both objected that the new foster care system involved far too much paperwork. Too many forms had to be completed, it took too long to process them all, and much of the information was repetitive and unnecessary. For example, if a child had to change placement in a short period of time, it was frustrating having to provide the same information all over again. We were told that the paperwork was a deterrent to referring children for placement at all and some children were being left in situations from which they really should have been removed. Almost all FAYS workers blamed the excessive paperwork associated with referral for their inability to implement reunification plans or formulate detailed case plans. The overall sentiment among FAYS workers and PSWs alike was that social work practice had become considerably more cumbersome and bureaucratic since the changeover. Even when regular contact with foster carers was maintained, there seemed to be little time to establish constructive working relationships with them or to work with children in placement. Although a lot more was being said about the need for case planning under they new system, FAYS workers conceded that few satisfactory case plans were being developed or implemented because of insufficient time and resources.

Declining practice standards

Foster care agencies repeatedly complained to us that, once a placement was made, FAYS workers were difficult to contact and many seemed undertrained in alternative care. FAYS workers accused PSWs of precisely the same things. CACU complained that placements seemed poorly planned by FAYS workers and PSWs alike. CACU reported numerous cases where placements were found without assessments being completed by FAYS workers, or where the foster care agencies had made insufficient effort to find the best possible placement. Placement Support Workers argued that such problems occurred because it simply took too long for FAYS and CACU staff to complete and pass on assessment and referral information. And even when the requisite information was passed on, PSWs complained that the information was usually inadequate to effect a suitable match between children and carers. Foster care workers also complained that FAYS workers were making unrealistic demands on their services – demands that FAYS itself had never been able to meet when it had provided foster care.

One thing on which all workers agreed, however, was that the range of placement options was severely restricted – as a consequence of which children were being forced to change placements too often, were placed too far away from families of origin or were not matched with suitable carers – and that many foster carers lacked the skills to provide adequate care. According to rural workers, these problems were particularly acute in country areas where the shortage of foster placements for adolescents was compounded by a dearth of alternatives to foster care. FAYS workers also expressed dissatisfaction with the shortage of placements for Aboriginal children, and with difficulties in placing siblings together. In around one-third of cases, Aboriginal children have to be placed with white families, or with foster families containing both Aboriginal and non-Aboriginal children (Barber, Delfabbro and Cooper 2000). Another common complaint was that the views of children were no longer being considered when placements were made. Although workers from metropolitan FAYS offices emphasized that these were not new problems, they believed that the situation had worsened in recent times because of deteriorating relationships between the agencies involved. The shortage of suitable carers was seen by most workers as probably the most fundamental cause of problems in the foster care system. Most workers also believed that the quality of carers was diminishing all the time. Foster care workers in particular believed that many good carers had been lost in the transition when FAYS and other agencies handed over their lists of foster carers. Foster care workers also expressed doubts about the quality of carers who transferred from FAYS to the foster care agencies. Most workers also lamented the lack of support now provided to carers by the state, and the fact that no concerted recruitment campaign had been conducted for years.

According to FAYS workers, foster carers were becoming less flexible all the time. Increasing numbers were refusing to take difficult children, refusing to take on reasonable parental responsibilities or refusing to take adolescents altogether. Some carers were also said to be poorly trained or unsuited to the task. Increasing numbers of carers seemed to have work commitments, with the result that some children were left unsupervised during the day. According to FAYS workers, good carers were being overused by the foster care agencies and few new carers were being recruited, in part because of the unnecessarily slow and bureaucratic process involved in registration. This was said to be a particular problem for relatives wishing to become carers. FAYS workers also expressed frustration about not being involved in carer training or support.

FAYS workers and PSWs expressed concern about the lack of clarity surrounding carers' entitlement to incidental costs. If, for example, children damaged or stole property from the carer's home, did FAYS or the foster care agency have responsibility to compensate the carer? Workers said that this issue was a common source of tension between carers and FAYS workers. They also pointed out that the problem extended to expenses in general. It was alleged in one FAYS group that some carers treated payments as a source of income which was applied to general household expenses to the detriment of the child's access to basic necessities such as new shoes and clothes, and school expenses. FAYS workers felt that clearer guidelines had to be developed to clarify the obligations of carers and the purpose of remuneration. Under existing arrangements, reimbursement was under the control of FAYS offices which were inconsistent in their policies and procedures.

Considerable concern was also expressed regarding special needs loadings (see Chapter 3). FAYS workers in both metropolitan and country areas and also CACU believed that the increase in the number of children being granted special loadings was unjustified. They argued that increased payments should not be used as a means of 'propping up placements'. A particular concern among FAYS workers in metropolitan offices was the apparent increase in the number of children being diagnosed with Attention Deficit Hyperactivity Disorder (ADHD) and sedated. It was alleged that some of this was motivated by the joint desires to control behaviour and attract a financial loading. CACU workers also said that foster care agencies sometimes seemed to value each child according to the number of subsidies and extra payments the child could attract. Some FAYS workers bluntly asserted that the shortage of placements was being used by the foster care agencies and carers to blackmail FAYS into applying unjustified loadings. Some of these workers also suspected that certain carers were not interested in achieving placement stability because of the financial incentives associated with very short-term placements. Specifically, carers who took children for only one week were paid more per child than those who looked after the same child for longer. Furthermore, those who were paid for respite placements were paid for a full week of care even if the child stayed for only a part of that week. By contrast, PSWs expressed little concern about the misuse of special loadings or incidental expenses, and complained only about the meagre amounts paid. They believed that carers were inadequately remunerated for their services and that FAYS was taking far too long to remit payments.

Coming the raw prawn

When Australians suspect that someone is trying to put one over on them, they will often protest with the colloquialism: 'Don't come the raw prawn with me, mate!' This time-honoured Australian expression captures perfectly the sentiment expressed by some of our focus group participants when discussing the state government's decision to outsource foster care to the non-government agencies. The workers in the foster care agencies were certainly in no doubt that they had been tossed a hot potato and that the government had been motivated in part by a wish to avoid responsibility for the looming disaster in alternative care (see Chapter 3 for a fuller discussion of this issue). Adding insult to injury in the eyes of these workers was what they saw as deliberate cost-cutting by FAYS, which based its contract price only on the direct costs of foster care services. Infrastructure and indirect costs, the foster care agencies alleged, had been ignored. While such complaints could be seen as self-serving, coming as they did from the foster care agencies, there was some degree of sympathy with these assertions within FAYS focus groups as well. As one FAYS worker put it: 'Nothing's changed; the problem's been outsourced, that's all.' FAYS workers, especially those involved in service delivery, often suggested that the non-government agencies had been most unwise to tender for the provision of foster care because the whole system had been in crisis for years and was manifestly underfunded. 'It was a trap', one FAYS worker told us, 'and they [the foster care agencies] fell for it.'

Not all of the FAYS workers were sympathetic to the predicament in which foster care agencies found themselves. Numerous FAYS workers took the view that the agencies had submitted tenders that boasted of the quality of their services and the agencies should be accountable for those claims. These workers regarded themselves as customers who had bought a product which came with certain claims and guarantees and, like purchasers of any other consumer goods or service, they were entitled to insist that the item should perform in accordance with the manufacturer's warranty. This attitude was referred to by some of the PSWs in our focus groups as a 'master–servant relationship', which they believed was a new and particularly odious characteristic of the foster care system. These PSWs complained that FAYS workers treated them like 'hired help' rather than partners in the service of children.

Summary of workers' focus groups

As this rather distressing litany of complaints illustrates, morale among government and non-government workers was very low following the outsourcing of foster care. After combing through the many hours of transcripts generated by these groups, it was difficult to find a single positive comment about the state of the system. Even more troubling was the apparent decline in working relationships across the sector as the various parties accused one another of causing the problems. Not surprisingly, then, one of the most common sentiments endorsed by FAYS, CACU and foster care workers alike was the need for improved relations between all of the parties in the system. In general, workers felt that social work practice had become excessively bureaucratic and inflexible as prescriptive job specifications and procedures manuals combined with excessive form-filling to drive out professional judgement and collaboration.

The views of carers

Since foster care workers themselves found the division of responsibilities between FAYS and foster care agencies unhelpful, it is hardly surprising that this issue also became a significant theme within the carer focus groups. One carer captured the mood of carer focus groups when she said:

> I think the difference was that in the past when you actually had [one unit] to work with, that supported you as a family . . . that worked

really well. But then when you go and you separate it, and you have [FAYS] who supports the child and you have the [foster care agency] who are there for the family, the two don't meet. I actually can't work out how you can separate child and family . . . As far as [FAYS] goes, I don't actually think that they give a damn about us as a family unit.

In general, then, the carers to whom we spoke were dissatisfied with the new foster care system. Most felt that insufficient research and planning had gone into it and that it had never been explained to carers why change was necessary. As in the workers' groups, the foster carers provided numerous examples of poor social work, difficulties with communication and consultation, and inconsistent case management practices. Indeed, there was so much consistency between workers' and carers' views that much of what has already been discussed in this chapter summarizes the carer focus groups as well.

Erosion of working relationships

The decline in constructive working relationships discussed in workers' focus groups was perhaps the most dominant preoccupation of the carer focus groups. According to some carers, one consequence of the demarcation between FAYS and PSW responsibilities was that carers were now being caught up in conflicts between workers. One carer described herself as 'the meat in the sandwich' in repeated conflicts between her PSW and the child's FAYS worker. The PSW would complain to the carer that she (the PSW) was being excluded from team decisions about the child, while the FAYS worker would complain that the PSW was incompetent and failing to do her job. All of the carers in our groups also confirmed the PSWs' allegation that carers were rarely provided with adequate information about the children in their care. Among the examples provided by carers were instances where children were delivered to the door of the house and all the carer was told was the child's name. More than one carer complained of chronically ill children being delivered without the necessary medication or even the information that the child was ill. According to the carers, such problems were symptomatic of their exclusion from case planning and the lack of consultation that characterizes the foster care system today. One carer told us that after caring for a child for five years she was telephoned by a FAYS worker and informed that the child would be reunified with his family of origin in four days' time. Until that moment, the carer had no idea that reunification was even being contemplated. The carer had naturally become attached to the child during his time in her care and she was very distressed by the manner of the separation. Another instance of this insensitivity to the relationship between carer and child was provided by a carer who told us:

I had a little boy that had to go to hospital. He nearly died ... I was told by the FAYS worker that my care stopped the minute I deposited him [the child] in the hospital and that I was not responsible for going in every day and night to visit him and that basically when he was due to come out of hospital, they would notify me and if my placement was still available he could come back, but that if they needed to place another child with me in the meantime, he might not come back at all.

Not surprisingly, then, a number of foster carers felt that they were neither valued as team members nor recognized for the parental care they provided. Indeed, this issue of needing to feel respected and valued by the statutory authority occupied much of our discussion time.

Inconsistent case management practices

Compounding the problem of inadequate consultation was a perception by some focus group participants that FAYS in particular operated both unilaterally and inconsistently in its management of cases. One significant way this was manifest was in decisions about the financial support of children. According to one carer, there seemed to be 'one set of rules for one person and another set of rules for another person'. This carer was referring to the fact that some District Centres provided financial support for various things where others did not. For example, some children were denied special needs loadings for conditions that had resulted in the maximum loading to other children. Carers also referred to inconsistencies and breaches of care standards, such as the supposed limit of three foster children in the one house, which was relaxed in some cases and rigidly applied in others. Of particular concern to some of the carers was the conduct of so-called 'special investigations', which are investigations of complaints made against carers by foster children. Not only did carers feel that extremely trivial complaints were treated as if they constituted abuse in care, but the method of investigation seemed to vary according to the whim of the investigating officer.

The challenging behaviour of children in care

A number of carers impressed on us that most of the children in foster care can be extremely difficult to deal with. There was no suggestion in the carer groups that the population was any worse under the new system but all carers were agreed that foster children placed great demands on carers' patience and parenting skills. One carer described her introduction to foster care this way: 'They brought her [the foster child] home to me with her hanging out of the car, the government car doors flying open. She gets out in my driveway and punches [person's name] in the face.' Numerous anecdotes like this were proffered by carers. One carer described what happened when she served a meal the child did not like: 'Called me all the "f__ing" things he could lay his tongue on. "I am not eating that f__ing shit" . . . Stormed around and smoked all my cigarettes and burnt things.' Carers frequently used the term 'overloaded' when referring to the way they felt, and more than one carer told us that they would rather not have children in their care who qualified for a special needs loading. This latter claim, of course, stands in marked contradiction of the allegation by some FAYS workers that *only* children who attract loadings are valued by carers and agencies.

Praise for individual workers

Although carers were undoubtedly critical of the foster care system as a whole, it should not be thought that they were universally negative about their experiences. There was considerable praise for certain individual workers whom carers clearly admired for their determination to provide the best possible service despite the systemic obstacles. 'With my FAYS worker, I've had nothing but 100 per cent support,' one carer told us. This carer went on to say that 'Anglicare also give me 100 per cent, whatever I want . . . They walk in my home . . . they put the coffee on, make the coffee for me if I am busy . . . Absolutely fantastic.' Almost all carers proffered at least one example like this of a worker or workers for whom they had great respect. A new carer told us:

> I ring up Anglicare and I get exactly what I want if I've got a problem. I ring up FAYS; I want a government car: it is there. If I've got a troublesome child, I ring them [FAYS] up and they send out counsellors for her. This is the truth. I go to the hospital to visit them, you know the children in hospital, and my FAYS worker sends me a little thank you and a posy of flowers . . . I don't know if I'm getting special treatment but I have been looked after fantastically. When it was my birthday last week, I got cards and gifts from all my FAYS workers . . . I feel valued, I feel like I am special.

Certain workers from the foster care agencies came in for similarly lavish praise: 'My Anglicare worker has been absolutely superb. She has been there twenty-four hours a day for me and my husband and my family.'

General discussion

Much of this chapter clearly makes for depressing reading. According to our focus group participants, morale among workers and foster carers is low, practice standards are inconsistent and declining, co-operation and even mutual respect are rarities and the whole system is under-resourced.

At the time of writing, efforts were being made by the purchasers and the providers of foster care to address some of these problems and to inject a greater degree of flexibility and common sense into the system. However, it is difficult to avoid the conclusion that the problems conveyed to us are symptomatic of the more fundamental policy failures canvassed in Chapter 3. And problems such as these cannot be overcome through goodwill alone. In 1997, the state moved to create a quasi-market in foster care, and this can only be achieved when conflicting interests are made to compete with one another. Prior to the adoption of the funder–purchaser–provider model described in Chapter 3, all parties could be seen as collaborators working towards a common cause, but the quasi-market requires a radical redefinition of the rules of the game. Under the funder–purchaser–provider model, the objective of the state purchaser is to minimize price and maximize service, whereas providers strive to maximize price and minimize service costs. As this chapter shows, the quasi-market has been spectacularly successful in pitting the parties' interests against one another and it has achieved this feat in a very short space of time. What this chapter also demonstrates, of course, is that competition itself comes at a price. Not that the quasi-market is the only factor lying behind the discontent within the foster care system. Years of government cost-cutting, the systematic closure of alternatives to family-based foster care and the changing demography of Australian society described in Chapter 3 have all played their part in straining the foster care system to breaking point.

As with all such focus group studies involving small, non-probability samples, it is not possible to make claims about the external validity of the findings reported in this chapter. On the other hand, the consistency and vehemence of the views that were put to us do inspire confidence that we have captured a substantial body of opinion among workers and carers. Bluntly, an air of pessimism now hangs over the entire sector. In the chapters that follow, we examine the progress of the most important people within this system: the children themselves. Ultimately, it is the progress and well-being of the children that should determine whether all this pessimism is justified.

Chapter 6

Background characteristics of children entering foster care

Introduction

During the last thirty years, there have been many studies that have detailed the needs and problems of children in foster care. Although studies have differed in the methodologies employed and the factors considered, the findings have generally been consistent. Children in foster care tend to obtain lower scores on most measures of psychosocial and physical well-being compared with normative populations of a similar age. Within foster care populations, there is a higher prevalence of disabilities and developmental difficulties (Coyne and Brown 1986; Hochstadt *et al.* 1987; Reed 1997); poorer educational outcomes (Blome 1997; Dubowitz *et al.* 1994; Heath, Colton and Aldgate 1994), conduct disorder and offending (Reid, Kagan and Schlosberg 1988); psychological problems such as hyperactivity, depression and anxiety, and difficulties in socialization (Klee and Halfon 1987). A substantial percentage of foster children are victims of abuse (Benedict *et al.* 1989; Courtney 1994; Hochstadt *et al.* 1987), and many come from family backgrounds with histories of intergenerational abuse, where parents have limited resources, parenting skills and social networks (Leifer, Shapiro and Kassem 1993). Given their background problems, it is not surprising that foster children are at significant disadvantage compared with other children, and that normative comparisons must be undertaken with considerable caution. Accordingly, a preferred approach, and one adopted in our own project, is to examine only within-sample changes; namely, how foster children fare over time relative to their own individual standards and competencies.

Although the central aim of much foster care research has been to determine how variations in placement experiences influence different children, much of it has been limited by a failure to appreciate the complex interaction between child and placement characteristics (Courtney 1993; Farmer 1996). Many of these problems are attributable not so much to any lack of understanding of the issues involved but to unsatisfactory methodological designs. As indicated in Chapter 4, the most significant limitation of these designs, and of cross-sectional designs in general, is that they tend to

over-sample children with longer placement histories. In studies of placement disruption, for example, conclusions have been drawn solely from
snapshot samples of children already in care, despite the fact that children
who are sampled from populations already in care are more likely to have
been in care longer, and to have experienced more placement changes than
other foster children not selected in this manner (Courtney 1994; Fanshel
and Shinn 1978; Fernandez 1999; Goerge 1990). Many correlational studies
also fail to consider the lack of independence between predictor variables,
or they attempt to infer causality on the basis of covariance, and they rarely
look for moderating or mediating variables. In studies that show a positive
relationship between the number of placement changes and behavioural
adjustment, for example, it may be tempting to conclude that placement
instability results in problematic behaviour. But, as pointed out in Chapter 4, if older children display more conduct problems and have also been in
care longer, it is hardly surprising that we should find associations between
challenging behaviours and placement disruption (Courtney 1994).

These concerns can be addressed in a number of ways. One of these is to
employ prospective longitudinal designs. Another is to place less emphasis
on group analyses that treat foster children as a homogeneous group, and
concentrate instead on individual difference variables and their relationship
with placement outcomes. This latter approach is implicit in Farmer's (1996)
distinction between two groups of children in the care system. She calls the
first group 'protected children' and she describes them as typically younger
children who come into care because of abuse and neglect. Farmer refers to
the second group as 'disaffected children' and these tend to be older children
who are placed in care, or remain in care, because of their own behavioural
and/or emotional problems. Thus, social work intervention with protected
children typically emphasizes the inability of parents to provide a safe, stable
and nurturing home environment, whereas the emphasis for the disaffected
children is on the children themselves, particularly their ability to control
their behaviour and adjust to the demands of everyday life.

Although useful in a descriptive sense, Farmer's analysis is limited in that
it provides little statistical basis for the dichotomy she has in mind. Instead,
her groups are based largely upon her clinical impressions of variables that
seem to go together. Nevertheless, there is empirical evidence from other
studies to suggest that her classification may well be valid. First, there is a
number of studies which show that placement instability, behavioural problems, truancy and offending behaviour are much more commonly observed
in older children (e.g., Aldgate and Hawley 1986; Bilson and Barker 1995;
Blome 1997; Colton and Williams 1997; Hochstadt *et al.* 1987; Hornby and
Collins 1981; Inglehart 1993; Lawder, Poulin and Andrews 1986; Palmer
1996; Schwab *et al.* 1986; Stone 1991), and that younger children are much
more likely to be in care as a result of parental factors such as abuse, neglect
and parental mental and physical ill-health (e.g., Farmer 1993; Fein and

Maluccio 1984; Gillespie, Byrne and Workman 1995; Inglehart 1994; Segal and Schwartz 1985). One aim of this chapter, therefore, is to examine the statistical validity of Farmer's classification system. Of particular interest in this context were the extent to which child characteristics influence the stability of placements; the types of placement available and the length of the legal order that applies. A second objective of this chapter is to examine the placement histories of the children in the study. This is important, not only because it describes how well these children have previously fared in the foster care system but also because it provides a baseline against which to compare subsequent placement changes observed in the larger tracking study.

In South Australia, as in other western jurisdictions, it is a policy requirement that children should experience as little disruption as possible when placed into foster care (Department for Family and Community Services 1996). A key intention of this policy is to provide children with the stability and continuity required for successful development and attachment. The policy is inspired by numerous studies showing that the frequency of placement change is inversely related to the probability of family reunification (e.g., Cantos, Gries and Slis 1997; Fanshel and Shinn 1978; Inglehart 1993; Pardeck 1983). Placement instability, or 'foster-care drift', as it is commonly called, has been a concerning feature of almost all western foster care systems for well over twenty years now, with teenage children being at greatest risk. In the United States, for example, Hornby and Collins (1981) found that 19 per cent of teenagers in care had six to ten previous placements, and 10 per cent had more than ten. More recently, Inglehart (1993) found that over a quarter of the adolescents placed in California had experienced four or more previous placements. Similar figures have also recently been reported by Palmer (1996). While many studies have examined the factors that predict placement instability, relatively little research has been undertaken to determine what effects placement instability has on child wellbeing. What research has been done, however, has found a link between placement instability, lower self-esteem and increased behavioural disturbance (e.g., Hicks and Nixon 1989; Inglehart 1993). In Chapter 10 we show that the relationship between instability and psychological adjustment is more complex than is often thought. Furthermore, a limitation of much existing research is that placement instability is not the only form of disruption experienced by children in foster care. Although changing foster parents may compromise the development of stable attachments, the total effect of any placement change will vary considerably depending upon the magnitude and nature of any attendant changes. Two additional factors which are particularly likely to compound the impact of placement change are whether or not the child also has to change schools, and the proximity of the child's birth family to the new placement. This problem of changing school has been highlighted by a number of researchers (Blome 1997; Combs-Orme,

Chernoff and Kager 1991). Blome found, for example, that 25 per cent of foster children changed school at least three times from the fifth grade until the end of high school compared with only 11 per cent of non-foster children. Despite this, there have been few attempts to gauge the effects of these changes on educational performance or the development of stable relationships with peers. Importantly, disrupting friendships is likely to cause considerable psychological distress in many children and a loss of interest in school; it may contribute to tension and placement breakdowns when children fail to complete homework or attend school. The issue of geographical dislocation is also seldom considered in foster care research despite being highly likely to influence the well-being of foster children. Clearly, the further a child is placed from either their birth family or their previous placement, the greater the probability of having to change schools, and the lower the likelihood of uninterrupted family contact.

The children's life circumstances and legal status

The demographic characteristics of the 235 children in our sample were described in Chapter 3 along with a summary of the baseline measures administered. Details of their intake levels of psychosocial adjustment will be presented in Chapter 7, and family contact in Chapter 8. In this chapter, we summarize the general circumstances and status of the children when they entered our study, including the factors that contributed to their being in care, their previous placement histories, their current placement status and their recent educational experiences.

Presenting problems

As indicated in Chapter 4, a number of issues and problems pertaining to the children and the circumstances of their placement were identified by social workers at intake. The first of these factors related to whether children had been the victims of any form of abuse. In addition, *child incapacity* was used to describe cases in which children had significant physical or mental health problems; *child mental health* referred to cases in which children were experiencing severe depression, suicidal ideation or self-destructive behaviours; *parental incapacity* was recorded when parents were in prison, had substance abuse problems or mental or physical illness; *family breakdown* referred to cases involving severe child–parent conflict; *child behaviour* identified children with problematic behaviours; and *homelessness* was recorded whenever children had nowhere to live. As indicated in Table 6.1, the most commonly reported factor at intake was some form of abuse, followed closely by parental incapacity brought on by substance abuse, mental ill-health or incarceration. Approximately one-third of the children had been subjected to at least one form of abuse, although fewer than a quarter of

Table 6.1 Significant problems identified by social workers at intake, n, (%)

	Total sample (n = 235)	Children changing placements[1] (n = 106)	Children entering the system (n = 129)
Active abuse			
Sexual abuse	27 (11.5)	16 (15.2)	11 (8.5)
Physical abuse	58 (24.7)	27 (25.7)	31 (24.0)
Emotional abuse	63 (26.8)	21 (20.0)	42 (32.6)
Unspecified abuse	13 (5.5)	13 (12.4)	n.a.
Parental problems			
Neglect	66 (28.1)	27 (25.7)	39 (16.6)
Parental incapacity	76 (32.3)	22 (22.9)	52 (40.3)
Child problems			
Child incapacity	49 (20.9)	26 (24.8)	23 (17.8)
Child mental health	46 (19.6)	20 (19.0)	26 (20.2)
Behavioural problems[2]	141 (60.0)	71 (67.6)	70 (54.3)
Family breakdown			
Family breakdown	32 (13.6)	12 (11.4)	20 (8.5)
Homelessness	8 (3.4)	0 (0.0)	8 (3.4)

Notes
1 Of the 100 already in care, 38 entered the study as a result of a confirmed placement breakdown; 37 had a suspected placement breakdown due to problematic behaviour, and the remaining 25 experienced a general placement change.
2 Also includes children classified with behavioural problems using the conduct disorder scale (mean item score > 1.0) and reports of substance abuse, offending, suspensions and problematic sexualized behaviours.

them had been subjected to serious physical or sexual abuse. Neglect was identified in almost a quarter of the cases, sometimes in conjunction with parental incapacity and homelessness. By contrast, relatively few children were referred because of a carer's inability to cope with the child's disability or developmental delay (*child incapacity*). Over half of the children entering care also had significant behavioural problems, although the prevalence of these characteristics did vary according to children's status at the time of placement. Proportion difference tests applied to the results in Table 6.1 showed that children entering the system for the first time were significantly more likely to be victims of emotional abuse, $z = 2.06$, $p < 0.05$, and to be in care because of parental incapacity, $z = 2.79$, $p < 0.01$ than were children who were merely changing placement. By contrast, children changing placement were significantly more likely to display behavioural problems, $z = 2.19$, $p < 0.05$.

The relationships between placement variables were assessed using a two-stage methodology. In the first stage, chi-square and correlational analyses

Table 6.2 Predictors of case status at intake

System variables	Beta	Wald	Odds-ratio
Number of placements			
Length of legal order	1.1	11.6***	2.87
64% of cases correctly classified			
Length of legal order			
Number of previous placements	0.1	16.3***	1.11
Family breakdown	−2.0	11.5**	0.13
Parental incapacity	−1.1	7.7**	0.32
Homelessness	2.9	6.1**	17.38
Sexual abuse	1.6	8.2**	5.04
Emotional abuse	−1.4	6.9**	0.32
76% of cases correctly classified			
Type of care			
Age	−0.2	3.9*	0.83
Offender	−1.2	4.7*	0.30
91% of cases correctly classified			

* $p < 0.05$, ** $p < 0.01$, *** $p < 0.001$

were conducted, as appropriate, to identify significant associations between variables. In the second stage, each binary variable, including placement type (1 = facility, 2 = foster care), length of legal order (1 = < 12 months, 2 = > 12 months), number of placements, offending (0 = no, 1 = yes) and problems identified at the time of the baseline placement (0 = doesn't apply, 1 = applies), was treated as a dependent measure in logistic regression analysis in which all significant univariate predictors of the dependent variable were entered as predictors.

As indicated in Table 6.2, many placement variables and case status variables were related. Children with longer-term orders experienced a greater number of previous placements, and longer orders were more likely to be applied to children who were homeless or were the victims of sexual abuse. On the other hand, family breakdown, parental incapacity and emotional abuse were more likely to be associated with a legal order of less than twelve months' duration. More specifically, family breakdown was associated with a 7.69 (1/0.13) times lesser likelihood of a long-term order, whereas parental incapacity and emotional abuse were both associated with a 3.13 (1/0.32) times reduced likelihood of a long-term placement. Children who had committed offences were 3.33 (1/0.33) times more likely to be placed into residential units, whereas each additional year (in age) was associated with a 1.20 (1/0.83) times greater likelihood of being in this type of arrangement. In summary, children who had been in care for longer periods and who had

Table 6.3 Predictors of problems at intake

Placement issue	Beta	Wald	Odds-ratio
Behaviour			
Age	0.2	20.1***	1.26
Gender	−1.2	12.8***	0.30
Number of placements	0.1	7.9*	1.08
Child mental health	1.4	6.7*	3.90
75% of cases correctly classified			
Child incapacity or disability			
Sexual abuse	0.9	4.1*	2.50
Neglect	1.2	11.7***	3.29
81% of cases correctly classified			
Parental incapacity			
Age	−0.2	25.7***	0.78
Length of legal order	−1.1	10.1***	0.32
73% of cases correctly classified			
Child mental health			
Gender	−1.2	9.4**	0.31
Age	0.2	9.2**	1.20
Number placements	0.1	4.5*	1.05
79% of cases correctly classified			

* $p < 0.05$, ** $p < 0.01$, *** $p < 0.001$

more severe problems were more likely to be bound by court orders, and older children with more problematic behaviours had a greater likelihood of being placed into more restrictive placement arrangements.

Although Table 6.3 replicates some of the information in Table 6.2, a number of additional trends can be discerned. Specifically, children with behavioural problems were more likely to be older, to be male, to have experienced a greater number of previous placements and to have mental health problems. Children with disabilities were more likely to be victims of sexual abuse or neglect. Mental health problems were more likely to be experienced by males, older children and those with longer placement histories. Finally, problems of parental incapacity tended to be more common in placements involving younger children and those who had short-term orders.

Placement history

Only 40 (16.7 per cent) of the children had not previously been placed into care compared with 194 (82.9 per cent) who had experienced at least one previous placement. Analysis of placement changes revealed high levels of

disruption. Forty-eight (20.5 per cent) children had 1 or 2 previous placements, 46 (19.7 per cent) had 3 to 5 previous placements, 41 (17.5 per cent)
had between 6 and 9 placements, and 55 (23.5 per cent) had been placed at
least 10 times previously. In fact, 15 of the children had experienced 20 or
more previous placements, including 2 who had lived in 34 separate foster
homes during their lifetime. Of those who had been placed before ($n = 194$),
123 (63 per cent) had been in care for less than twelve months in total, 42
(22 per cent) had been in placement for at least three years, and the remaining 30 (15 per cent) had been in placement between one and three years.
Half of those who had previously been in care (i.e., 50 per cent of 194) were
changing placements at the time they were referred into our study.

Educational disruption

The results showed that 182 (77 per cent) of the children were attending
school at the time of the survey and that, of these, 83 (45 per cent) had to
change school as a result of the new placement. Furthermore, there was a
significant association between current school change and the number of
changes that had occurred in the previous twelve months, χ^2 (2) = 60.52,
$p < 0.001$. Thirty-seven (45 per cent) of those who changed school for the new
placement had already changed school at least once in the previous twelve
months, with 12 children having done so 5 or more times before. A logistic
regression analysis, controlling for geographical distance, was conducted to
identify the child and placement characteristics that predicted school changes.
Apart from distance, age was the only significant factor which predicted
school changes, with each unit increase in age associated with a 1.18 times
greater likelihood of changing school. By contrast, each increase on the
geographical distance scale (see below) led to a 3.45 times greater likelihood
of a school change. The origin of the child (country versus metropolitan)
did not influence school changes. Interestingly, when this analysis was
undertaken separately for children already in care and those coming into
care, the results held only for the children already in care. This suggests
that disruption of schooling is more likely to be a problem for older children with a longer placement history.

Geographical dislocation

Table 6.4 shows how far children were placed from their nearest birth family
member (parents or primary caregiver). As indicated, 85 (36 per cent) were
placed within 10 km of their families, but a greater number – 102 (43 per
cent) – were placed more than 20 km away. Further analyses revealed significant associations between geographical location and gender, with 53 per
cent of boys being placed more than 20 km from their homes compared
with only 33 per cent of girls, χ^2 (4) = 14.27, $p < 0.01$. Location was also

Table 6.4 Proximity of placement (km) to nearest birth family member, *n*, (%)

Very close (< 5)	43 (18)
Quite close (5–10)	42 (18)
Slightly remote (11–20)	41 (17)
Quite remote (21–50)	48 (20)
Very remote (51+)	54 (23)

associated with school changes, χ^2 (4) = 64.22, $p < 0.001$, with 75 per cent of those who were placed 21 km or further from their home having to change school. Not surprisingly, geographical dislocation was greater for children in country areas than in the metropolitan area, χ^2 (4) = 12.27, $p < 0.01$, with 62 per cent of country children being placed more than 20 km from home compared with only 42 per cent of metropolitan children.

Sub-groups within the sample

To assist in the process of identifying groups within the sample, a cluster analysis was undertaken. Included in this analysis were demographic characteristics, placement history and intake problems. Data were analysed initially using a hierarchical clustering procedure to determine the appropriate number of clusters (Hair *et al.* 1995). Using squared Euclidian distance as the similarity measure, several separate analyses were conducted to ascertain the stability of the cluster solution in relation to variations in the cluster method, including the centroid method and Ward's method. As all solutions were almost identical, only the results using the centroid method with squared Euclidian distance are reported here. Initially, the results suggested a three-cluster solution. However, since the third cluster contained only three cases and resembled the second cluster anyway, a two-cluster solution was chosen.

To identify the characteristics of the two clusters, a non-hierarchical or K-means cluster analysis was undertaken. This analysis showed that the two clusters (Cluster 1, $n = 132$; Cluster 2, $n = 103$) could be distinguished in terms of significant mean differences on eight variables. These variables and the magnitude of the differences are presented in Table 6.5, which summarizes the mean scores for interval-level variables (age) and the proportion of individuals in each cluster possessing each of the binary characteristics.

Table 6.5 shows clear differences in the composition of the two clusters. The first group of children (Cluster 1) tended to be male, were older and had behavioural problems. By contrast, Cluster 2 consisted of younger children who were more likely to be in care because of parental incapacity or neglect.

Table 6.5 Differences between means of variables defining the two clusters

	Cluster 1 (n = 132)	Cluster 2 (n = 103)	F-value
Gender (M = 1, F = 2)	1.55	1.40	5.65*
Age	13.35	7.44	647.72***
Behavioural problems	0.70	0.47	14.44**
Parental incapacity	0.20	0.49	24.07***
Neglect	0.20	0.38	9.26**

Notes
1   All variables scored (0 = issue did not apply, 1 = issue applied), except age and gender.
2   Percentages for binary variables were significantly different according to chi-squared tests.
3   $* p < 0.05$, $** p < 0.01$, $*** p < 0.001$

General discussion

The results presented in this chapter were generally consistent with Farmer's (1993) distinction between 'disaffected' and 'protected' children. The disaffected children in our sample were almost always teenagers who had been placed into care as a result of behavioural problems such as truancy, offending and aggression, whereas protected children were typically under ten years old and had been placed because their parents were unable to provide adequate care. In some cases the parents of protected children had suffered mental or physical illnesses requiring hospitalization, and in other cases the parents were affected by serious substance abuse or were convicted offenders. Consistently with previous overseas studies (e.g., Benedict et al. 1989; Benedict and White 1991; Hudson, Nutter and Galaway 1992; Klee and Halfon 1987), many disaffected children also displayed mental health problems such as depression, anxiety and suicidal ideation. This contrasted with the younger, protected children who were more likely to be diagnosed with neurological disorders such as attention deficit disorder and developmental delay. We will need to return to this distinction between protected and disaffected children in later chapters because of the very different placement outcomes experienced by the two groups. As we shall see, the poorest outcomes in foster care tend to be concentrated within the disaffected population, and it is this group which most urgently requires a wider range of placement options than is currently available.

Somewhat surprisingly, the results of our analysis of intake characteristics revealed no significant relationship between age and placement history. Although it was expected that older children would have a longer placement history with a greater number of placement changes (cf. Courtney 1995a; Hornby and Collins 1981; Farmer 1993), many of the children with the highest numbers of placement changes were under twelve years of age. A likely

explanation for this finding is that adolescents with the most disrupted placement histories tend to leave the system before they turn eighteen years of
age. This would occur because social workers come to the conclusion that
conventional family-based foster care is simply inappropriate for adolescents with a history of placement disruption, and so make arrangements for
these children to move into institutional care or independent living. Despite
the absence of such children from our sample, the data show that foster
children experience considerable disruption when placed into care. In addition to the remarkable number of placement changes already experienced by
our sample, the children also endured considerable disruption to their schooling and family life when referred into foster care. Almost half of the sample
were forced to change school because of the referral, and 43 per cent were
placed more than 20 km from their nearest birth family member. The extent
of this disruption varied, of course, depending upon the location of the
placement and certain background child characteristics. In particular, school
changes were more likely in the rural areas and for older children, again
highlighting the trend towards less desirable placement options for older
children.

Taken together, then, these findings suggest that many of the children
entering the foster care system are already accustomed to frequent placement
movements, school changes and geographical separation from birth parents.
In the next chapter, we examine what happened to this sample of children in
the two years following this referral.

Chapter 7

The progress and satisfaction of children in care

Introduction

Foster children are in an invidious position: most of them have a home somewhere but for a variety of reasons they must move out of it and live with strangers until some other adult works out what to do next. The dependence and powerlessness of children in this predicament are obvious, and the obstacles to their development seem formidable. On the face of it, it seems unreasonable to expect foster children to slip quietly and happily into placement, at least in the short to medium term. The purpose of this chapter is to investigate the extent to which the foster children in our sample did adjust to care. In the first part of the chapter, we present the children's placement movements and psychosocial well-being at each stage of the study. As previously indicated (see Chapter 3), Stage 1 spanned the period from intake to four months, Stage 2 from four to eight months, Stage 3 from eight months to one year, and Stage 4 from one to two years. Each section begins with a diagrammatic presentation of placement movements, in which a stable placement has been operationally defined as a single address throughout the period. An unstable placement, then, was one where a child had to change placement at least once in the period.

In addition to placement stability and psychosocial adjustment, this chapter also presents the feedback of foster children on their placements. A key tenet of the United Nations Convention on the Rights of the Child is that children's views should be taken into account in any decision that is likely to affect their well-being or position in life (Gilligan 2000). As previously indicated (see Chapters 1 and 4), this view now features strongly in alternative care policies around the world. Despite this, few systematic attempts have been made to obtain information regarding children's satisfaction with care. One explanation for this may be that this kind of research is inherently difficult for logistical reasons (see Gilbertson and Barber 2002). The requirement in many jurisdictions to obtain consent from foster carers, parents, service providers and children inevitably limits access to many children in care. Furthermore, doubts have also been raised about the extent to which foster children are likely to express their true feelings about foster homes. The approach taken in this study was to limit our interviews to a sub-sample which was broadly representative of the overall sample and to use interviewers who were manifestly unconnected with the foster care system.

Placement destinations

Of the 235 children in our sample who were referred into foster care, 109 (46 per cent) were still in care two years later. This section reports on the placement movements between intake and each follow-up point until termination of data collection.

Four-month follow-up

The intake sample can be divided into three groups: (1) new referrals to care ($n = 40$); (2) those who were returning to care after going home from a previous placement ($n = 89$); and (3) those in care who needed to change placements ($n = 106$). Figure 7.1 identifies these three groups and describes the placement status of the intake sample ($n = 235$) at the four-month point.

Figure 7.1 shows that 35 (15 per cent) of the 235 children who entered care at intake had returned home by the four-month follow-up point after a single foster placement. Another 72 (32 per cent) were assigned to a single placement which remained intact for the entire period, and 5 (2 per cent) ended up outside of the care system, but did not go home. The remaining 123 (53 per cent) children changed placement at least once during the period. After changing placements at least once, a further 24 (20 per cent) returned home by the end of the period, 92 (75 per cent) were still in care, and 7 (6 per cent) were in custody, were in independent living or were unaccounted for.

Table 7.1 shows that placement status at the four-month follow-up varied depending on the group to which the children belonged at intake. Specifically, proportion difference tests showed that new referrals were significantly more likely to return home than the other two groups, $z = 3.99$, $p < 0.01$.

Eight-month follow-up

Figure 7.2 presents the placement movements of children who were in care at the four-month point and again at the eight-month follow-up point. It shows a relatively high rate of placement stability over the period for children who began the period at home. At eight months, 52 (88 per cent) of the children at home at the start of the period remained there at least until the eight-month point, and a further 2 (3 per cent) returned home after a short period in care. Only 5 (8 per cent) of the children who started the period at home ended up in care at eight months, although 4 of them experienced

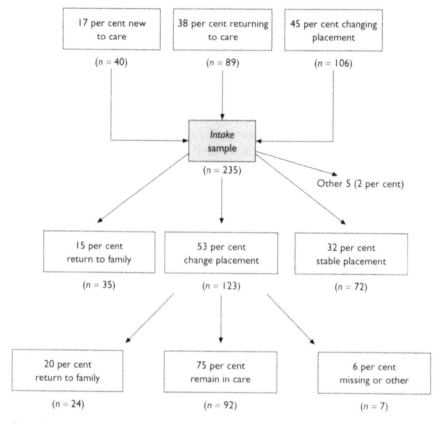

Figure 7.1 Placement changes from intake to four months

Table 7.1 Status at follow-up by origin of child, n, (%)

	New to care (n = 40)	Returning to care (n = 89)	Changing placement (n = 106)
Returned home	20 (50.0)	29 (32.6)	10 (9.4)
Stable foster placement	11 (27.5)	30 (33.3)	35 (33.0)
Unstable foster placement	7 (17.5)	31 (34.8)	54 (50.9)

placement instability after returning to care. Of the 72 children who had found a stable placement by the four-month point, 12 (17 per cent) returned home by the eight-month point, and a further 49 (68 per cent) remained in placement throughout the period. On the other hand, 10 (14 per cent) of the children who had previously been stable experienced placement change

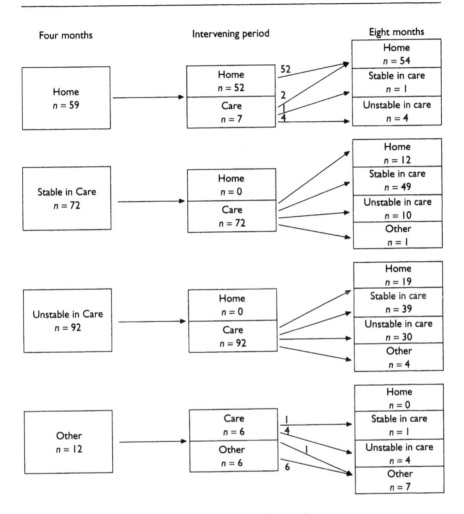

Figure 7.2 Placement movements from four to eight months

between the four- and eight-month points. Of the 92 children who had experienced placement instability during the earlier period, 39 (42 per cent) settled down in this period and remained in one foster home, while a further 19 (21 per cent) went home. However, fully one-third of this sub-group ($n = 30$) had still not found a stable home after eight months but continued to bounce around the foster care system. Finally, of the 12 children who began the second period in 'other' arrangements, primarily residential care, 7 (58 per cent) continued in those arrangements at the eight-month point, 4 (33 per cent) went back into foster care but experienced at least one placement breakdown during the period, and only 1 (8 per cent) found a stable foster home.

Twelve-month follow-up

Figure 7.3 presents the placement movements of children who were in care at the eight-month point and again at the one-year point. Children who began the period at home remained quite stable, with 81 (95 per cent) of the 85 who started the period at home remaining there throughout. Of the others, 2 (2 per cent) went into an unstable foster arrangement, and 2 (2 per cent) ended up in supervised accommodation. Of the 90 children who began the period stable in care, 55 (61 per cent) remained that way throughout this period as well, and a further 7 (8 per cent) returned home. On the other hand, 27 (30 per cent) had to move out of their placements, mainly to another foster home ($n = 25$). Of the 49 children who had been unstable in care during the former period, 28 (57 per cent) settled into a single placement in this period and 3 (6 per cent) went home. Sixteen (33 per cent) of the previously unstable children continued to be unstable during this period also, and 2 (4 per cent) moved out of foster care altogether. Finally, almost all of the 11 children who began the period in something other than a foster home (mainly residential care) were still outside of the foster care system at the end of the period.

Two-year follow-up

Figure 7.4 presents placement movements between the one- and two-year follow-up points. The diagram shows that 80 (87 per cent) of the children who were home at the one-year point were still there at two years, with the remainder being in either 'other' arrangements (mainly youth shelters or residential care) (9 per cent) or in unstable foster homes (3 per cent). Of the 83 children who had been stable in foster care at the one-year point, 50 (60 per cent) remained that way at the two-year point, and a further 10 (12 per cent) returned home. However, 20 (24 per cent) of the previously stable children were required to change placement at least once during the period. Forty-three children had been unstable in foster care at one year, and 26 (60 per cent) of them remained that way at the two-year point. Only 9 (21 per cent) of the unstable group had found their way into a stable foster placement, and a further 5 (12 per cent) had gone home.

Summary of placement destinations

Table 7.2 presents a summary of placement destinations at the end of each follow-up point. Throughout the study period, then, the most common placement destination was either in stable or unstable foster care, with a sharp decline in the number of unstable placements after the initial four-month period. The least desirable placement type, unstable in care, occurred in almost 40 per cent of cases during Stage 1 before settling on a rate of approximately

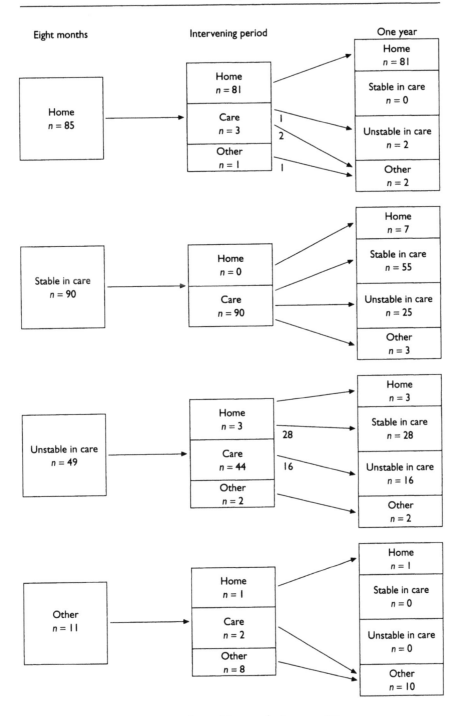

Figure 7.3 Placement movements from eight months to one year

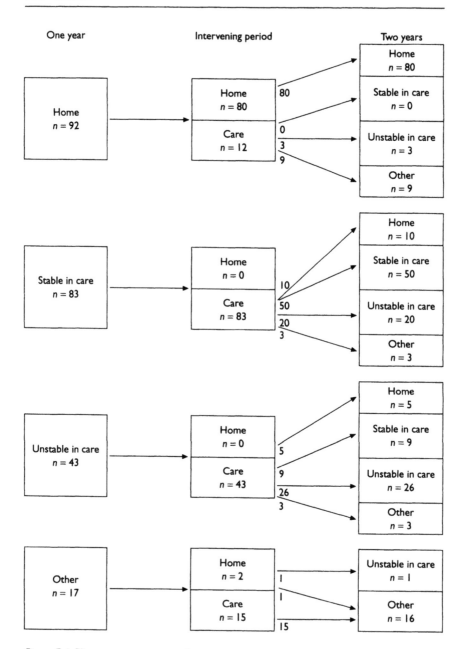

Figure 7.4 Placement movements from one to two years

Table 7.2 Status summary at each follow-up point, n (%) (n = 235)

	Went home	Stable in care	Unstable in care	Other
At 4 months	59 (25.1)	72 (30.6)	92 (39.1)	12 (5.1)
At 8 months	85 (36.2)	90 (38.3)	49 (20.9)	11 (4.7)
At 12 months	92 (39.1)	83 (35.3)	43 (18.3)	17 (7.2)
At 2 years	95 (40.4)	59 (25.1)	50 (21.3)	31 (13.1)

Table 7.3 Reasons for placement change at each follow-up point, n, (%)

	0–4 mths	4–8 mths	8–12 mths	1–2 years
Number of placement moves	445	166	164	235
Reason for move				
Only ever intended to be short-term	216 (48.5)	54 (32.5)	44 (26.8)	53 (22.6)
Child's behaviour	79 (17.8)	31 (18.7)	53 (32.3)	60 (25.5)
Child wanted to leave	9 (4.2)	7 (4.2)	0 (0.0)	3 (1.3)
More suitable option found	16 (3.6)	31 (18.7)	27 (16.5)	68 (28.9)
Reunification with family	62 (13.9)	25 (15.1)	10 (6.1)	9 (3.8)
Child ran away	13 (2.9)	6 (3.6)	8 (4.8)	7 (3.0)
Foster carer couldn't cope	32 (7.2)	7 (4.2)	6 (3.7)	0 (0.0)
Child was arrested	2 (0.9)	0 (0.0)	10 (6.1)	29 (12.3)
Moved to independent living; other	16 (7.5)	5 (3.0)	6 (3.6)	6 (2.4)

20 per cent for the remainder of the study. Table 7.2 also shows that, at the end of the first study period, around a quarter of the sample had returned home, with that number rising to one-third and eventually to around 40 per cent by the end of the period. Table 7.3 presents the total number of placement moves within each study period together with a breakdown of the reasons behind the moves.

Table 7.3 shows that, after the second study period, the prevalence of the child's putatively disruptive behaviour increased as an explanation for placement change. Another noteworthy feature of Table 7.3 is the very large number of placements that were only ever intended to be short-term, particularly during Stage 1 of the study. While there are no doubt many good reasons why it may be necessary to make short-term placements from time to time, it is obviously preferable to avoid such arrangements wherever possible and to seek more stable foster homes from the outset.

Psychosocial outcomes

Turning now to psychosocial adjustment, this section presents results of standardized assessments at intake and at every follow-up point thereafter.

Table 7.4 Means, (SD) of CBC sub-scales, up to four months

	Intake	4 months	t-value	Effect size (d)
Conduct				
Damaged property	0.50 (0.64)	0.40 (0.67)	1.88	0.15
Destroyed property	0.68 (0.67)	0.48 (0.72)	3.01[2]	0.29
Disobedient at school	0.92 (0.75)	0.84 (0.76)	1.07	0.11
Lied or cheated	1.13 (0.69)	0.97 (0.76)	2.41[1]	0.22
Stole things	0.49 (0.70)	0.40 (0.66)	1.53	0.13
Physical attacks	0.52 (0.69)	0.41 (0.63)	1.94	0.17
Mean score	0.71 (0.51)	0.59 (0.52)	3.02[2]	0.21
Hyperactivity				
Couldn't concentrate	1.33 (0.72)	1.17 (0.81)	2.26[1]	0.21
Couldn't sit still	1.00 (0.79)	0.93 (0.82)	1.21	0.09
Distractible	1.20 (0.72)	1.02 (0.79)	2.89[2]	0.24
Mean score	1.17 (0.66)	1.00 (0.70)	3.08[2]	0.28
Emotionality				
Unhappy, sad or depressed	1.21 (0.59)	1.14 (0.61)	1.14	0.12
Not as happy as other children	1.21 (0.60)	1.11 (0.69)	1.43	0.16
Nervous and tense	0.94 (0.76)	0.86 (0.75)	1.14	0.11
Too fearful or anxious	0.81 (0.73)	0.78 (0.64)	< 1	0.04
Worried a lot	1.11 (0.65)	0.95 (0.72)	2.22[1]	0.23
Mean score	1.07 (0.53)	0.93 (0.51)	2.80[1]	0.19
Social adjustment	3.00 (0.51)	2.96 (0.41)	< 1	0.04

Notes
1   0.05
2   0.01

Four-month follow-up

Table 7.4 presents mean item scores on the CBC sub-scales and social adjustment for the children who were in care at intake and first follow-up ($n = 164$). Within-samples analysis of conduct scores revealed an improvement in behaviour from intake to four-month follow-up. Analysis of individual conduct items showed that the change in overall score was due to a significant reduction in two of the six items, with children being less likely to destroy property or lie and cheat once they had been in care for four months. Similarly, there was a significant reduction in overall hyperactivity, due in this case to two of the three items: concentration problems and distractibility. Finally, the change in overall emotionality score was due to improvement in one of the five items – 'worried a lot'. Taken together, then, these analyses suggest that children in care for four months were generally better behaved, less agitated and less worried than they had been at intake.

Table 7.5 School performance and adjustment at intake and follow-up, *n*, (%)
(follow-up figures in bold, negative items in italics)

	Often	Sometimes	Rarely	Never
Has not completed homework or	*21 (25.6)*	*35 (42.7)*	*16 (19.5)*	*10 (12.2)*
set work	**16 (19.5)**	**34 (41.5)**	**9 (11.0)**	**13 (15.9)**
Has been attentive in class	29 (30.9)	48 (51.1)	16 (17.0)	1 (1.2)
	33 (35.1)	**38 (40.4)**	**12 (12.7)**	**3 (3.6)**
Has been disruptive in class	*27 (22.9)*	*41 (34.7)*	*14 (11.9)*	*16 (13.6)*
	19 (16.1)	**50 (42.4)**	**19 (16.1)**	**20 (16.9)**
Has refused to take part in activities	*11 (13.4)*	*31 (37.8)*	*16 (19.5)*	*24 (29.3)*
	9 (11.0)	**20 (24.4)**	**13 (15.6)**	**33 (40.2)**
Has been well-organized	21 (26.9)	20 (25.6)	28 (35.9)	9 (11.5)
	17 (21.8)	**29 (37.2)**	**19 (24.4)**	**6 (7.7)**
Has been interested in studies	26 (29.2)	43 (48.3)	16 (18.0)	4 (4.5)
	27 (30.3)	**43 (48.3)**	**11 (12.4)**	**3 (3.4)**
Has been disciplined by staff	*31 (33.7)*	*41 (44.6)*	*9 (9.8)*	*11 (11.6)*
	23 (25.0)	**38 (41.3)**	**10 (10.9)**	**8 (8.7)**
Has produced work of a good	18 (21.2)	43 (50.6)	18 (21.2)	6 (7.1)
standard	**21 (24.7)**	**38 (44.7)**	**11 (12.9)**	**6 (7.1)**
Has been late to class	*18 (22.5)*	*15 (17.6)*	*9 (11.3)*	*38 (47.6)*
	7 (8.8)	**14 (16.5)**	**10 (12.5)**	**33 (41.3)**
Has wagged (skipped) school	*16 (17.0)*	*11 (11.7)*	*6 (6.4)*	*61 (64.9)*
	6 (6.4)	**9 (9.6)**	**10 (10.6)**	**62 (66.0)**

Not surprisingly, however, assessments of effect sizes based on a comparison of mean difference scores and the standard deviations (Cohen 1992) revealed that the effects (d) over such a short period of time were small for all comparisons (i.e., < 0.30).

Table 7.5 indicates that a substantial number of children who remained in care for at least four months were experiencing significant problems in school at intake. Approximately one-quarter were often disruptive in class and were not completing set work, over a third were often disciplined by staff members and nearly a third were skipping school often or sometimes. Between one in five and one in three children were reported at intake as rarely or never being attentive in class, interested in their studies or producing work of 'a good standard'. Encouragingly, results showed some improvement in performance at school over the period. McNemar change tests were used to compare the relative percentage of children in the often and sometimes groups for each item compared with the percentage in the rarely and never categories. This procedure showed that children were significantly less likely to skip school at follow-up (29 per cent at intake versus 16 per cent at follow-up, $p < 0.05$), or to refuse to take part in school activities (51 per cent at intake versus 35 per cent at follow-up, $p < 0.05$). On the other hand, there was no significant improvement in how much interest children were showing in their studies, in the quality of work produced, level of organization, or general attentiveness.

A more objective measure of school adjustment can be derived by comparing the rate of school suspensions and exclusions at intake and follow-up. Sixty of the children in receipt of care throughout the study period had been suspended at least once in the twelve months prior to the study ($M = 0.95$, $SD = 1.94$) for a mean duration of fourteen days, and nine had been excluded ($M = 0.05$, $SD = 0.24$). During the first follow-up period, 26 children were suspended, with 8 having been suspended on three or more occasions. Each suspension was for approximately two to seven days. There were also 6 exclusions, with 4 of these children not returning to school at all. An approximate suspension rate can be calculated by dividing the pre-placement mean by 3 to give mean suspension rate per quarter of 0.32. This compares with 0.17 for the first follow-up period using the same logic. Thus, both social worker ratings and suspensions data suggest a decrease in problematic school behaviours during the first four months in placement.

Results at the four-month point are therefore consistent with the conclusion that foster placement tends to be accompanied by short-term improvements in conduct disorder, hyperactivity and emotional disorder. There was also a statistically significant improvement in the children's attendance and participation at school, and this improvement was reflected in a lower rate of school exclusions after the children came into care. It must be emphasized, of course, that, in the absence of an adequate control condition, improvements in behaviour and well-being cannot be attributed to foster placement itself. Among the more obvious threats to the internal validity of this conclusion in the present instance is child maturation. Whatever the explanation, however, it is encouraging none the less to find that psychosocial adjustment generally improves in foster care.

Eight-month follow-up

Nelson, Singer and Johnsen (1978) note that improvements in the child's functioning on entering care are likely to be short-lived, as most children can be expected to conform at least temporarily to the behavioural expectations of a new setting. On the contrary, the findings presented in Table 7.6 suggest that adjustment scores of the 139 children still in care at the eight-month follow-up point continued to exceed intake levels. Because of the large amount of missing data in relation to educational items for each child the longer the study went on, measures of psychosocial adjustment beyond four months in care had to be restricted to CBC and social adjustment scores. Missing data also precluded analysis of individual CBC items.

A one-way repeated measures analysis of variance, with Time as the repeated factor, was applied to each of CBC sub-scale score. This procedure

Table 7.6 Means, (SD) of CBC sub-scales, 0–8 months

	Intake	4 months	8 months
Conduct disorder (n = 117)	0.72 (0.50)	0.64 (0.54)	0.55 (0.48)
Hyperactivity (n = 112)	1.20 (0.65)	1.03 (0.73)	1.11 (0.69)
Emotionality (n = 117)	1.05 (0.48)	0.95 (0.51)	0.84 (0.56)
Social adjustment (n = 124)	2.97 (0.51)	2.97 (0.42)	3.04 (0.43)

revealed a significant main effect of Time for conduct disorder, $F(2, 114) = 5.09$, $p < 0.01$, which took the form of a significant negative linear trend, $F(1, 115) = 10.27$, $p < 0.01$. Fisher Least Significant Difference (LSD) tests applied to this result showed that conduct scores at eight months were significantly lower than at intake ($p < 0.05$) but not than at four months. Similarly, there was a significant improvement in emotionality scores across time, $F(2, 114) = 8.07$, $p < 0.001$, again characterized by a significant negative linear trend, $F(1, 115) = 13.37$, $p < 0.001$. A Fisher test revealed that emotionality scores at eight months were significantly lower than at intake ($p < 0.05$) but not than at four months. The same analyses revealed no significant change in hyperactivity or social adjustment scores from intake to eight months, although the change for hyperactivity was close to significance ($p = 0.07$) and in the same direction as conduct and emotionality. Effect size analyses indicated that the effect for conduct was small ($d = 0.35$), and the difference between intake and eight-month scores for emotionality was moderate ($d = 0.40$).

Twelve-month follow-up

Although the prevalence of missing values at any one follow-up point was not excessive (approximately 15 per cent of cases), the accumulation of missing values across time combined with listwise deletion in repeated measures analysis meant that it was not feasible or useful to compare all four sets of data available at twelve months. Instead, pairwise comparisons were conducted to ascertain whether improvements in adjustment observed at eight months were also evident when comparing twelve-month scores with intake scores (Table 7.7). Repeated measures analysis revealed that conduct disorder

Table 7.7 Means, (SD) of CBC sub-scales, eight to twelve months

	Intake	12 months
Conduct disorder (n = 112)	0.72 (0.50)	0.59 (0.48)
Hyperactivity (n = 108)	1.20 (0.64)	1.10 (0.69)
Emotionality (n = 111)	1.07 (0.48)	0.81 (0.55)
Social adjustment (n = 117)	2.94 (0.54)	2.83 (0.60)

scores had indeed improved at twelve months compared with those at intake, $F(1, 110) = 5.00$, $p < 0.05$. The same trend was observed for emotionality, $F(1, 109) = 17.42$, $p < 0.001$, but not for hyperactivity, $F(1, 106) < 1$, which remained relatively stable over time. Effect size analyses showed that the improvement in conduct scores could be classified as small ($d = 0.27$), whereas the improvement in emotionality constituted a moderate effect ($d = 0.51$). Overall, then, the general improvements in pychosocial well-being observed over the period up to eight months were maintained after twelve months in care.

Two-year follow-up

The two-year series of analyses (Table 7.8) was undertaken in the same manner as those completed for the eight-month follow-up period, except that the interval between measurement points this time was extended to twelve months. Thus, the analyses for twelve months were extended by comparing psychosocial adjustment scores recorded at two years with those obtained at twelve months and at intake. Naturally this comparison involved only those children still in care after two years. The total number was therefore 109, although data were not available at some follow-up points for some children, thereby reducing the overall numbers for the analyses that follow.

A repeated measures ANOVA revealed a significant Time main effect for conduct, $F(2, 87) = 6.211$, $p < 0.01$, and also for emotionality, $F(2, 86) = 4.89$, $p < 0.01$, both of which displayed significant negative linear trends: $F(1, 86) = 11.31$, $p < 0.001$ (for conduct disorder), $F(1, 86) = 7.94$, $p < 0.01$ (for emotionality). Fisher LSD post-hoc tests applied to these results identified the same phenomenon in both cases. Scores at both twelve months and two years were significantly lower than at intake, but scores at two years were no different from those at twelve months. In other words, initial improvements in psychosocial well-being observed soon after placement into foster care were maintained after two years in care. Again, there was no significant change in hyperactivity, $F(2, 83) < 1$, for the sample as a whole.

Table 7.8 Means, (SD) of CBC sub-scales, one to two years

	Intake	I year	2 years
Conduct disorder ($n = 89$)	0.80 (0.47)	0.65 (0.51)	0.60 (0.53)
Hyperactivity ($n = 86$)	1.27 (0.58)	1.16 (0.67)	1.17 (0.66)
Emotionality ($n = 88$)	1.07 (0.45)	0.88 (0.54)	0.90 (0.57)
Social adjustment ($n = 93$)	2.95 (0.58)	2.78 (0.60)	2.71 (0.53)

Psychosocial outcomes based on cluster classification at intake

A second series of analyses compared the long-term psychosocial adjustment of children initially classified within the 'protected' and 'disaffected' clusters described in Chapter 6. Scores obtained at intake, twelve months and two years (Table 7.9) were compared using a 2 (Cluster) × 3 (Time) repeated measures ANOVA. In general, the results revealed few significant differences between the two clusters. For conduct disorder, there was only a significant main effect of Time, $F (2, 174) = 5.41$, $p < 0.01$, involving a trend towards improvement in both groups over time.

For hyperactivity, there was no main effect of Time, but there was a significant main effect of Cluster, $F (1, 84) = 6.83$, $p < 0.01$. As indicated by Table 7.9, this result is due to lower scores within the protected group at twelve months and at two years. A similar analysis applied to emotionality showed that there was a general decrease in emotionality scores across time in both groups, $F (2, 172) = 4.85$, $p < 0.01$, but no other significant effects.

In short, although it might be expected that the disaffected group of children would experience relatively poorer psychosocial outcomes over time, the one difference that was observed actually favoured the disaffected group. More specifically, both groups experienced similar changes in conduct disorder and emotionality scores, but hyperactivity worsened in the protected group. There are at least two reasons why this might have been so. The first is simply that some of the children in the protected sample progressed from late childhood into early adolescence over the life of the study, so the observed increase in hyperactivity could have been due to maturation. Secondly, some

Table 7.9 The psychological adjustment of protected and disaffected children after two years in care, means, (SD)

	Protected cluster (n = 52)	Disaffected cluster (n = 57)
Conduct disorder		
Baseline	0.79 (0.43)	0.81 (0.50)
At 12 months	0.74 (0.52)	0.58 (0.50)
At 2 years	0.61 (0.53)	0.60 (0.54)
Hyperactivity		
Baseline	1.32 (0.49)	1.24 (0.65)
At 12 months	1.33 (0.59)	1.02 (0.71)
At 2 years	1.39 (0.53)	1.00 (0.70)
Emotionality		
Baseline	1.11 (0.47)	1.04 (0.43)
At 12 months	0.94 (0.55)	0.84 (0.53)
At 2 years	0.93 (0.59)	0.89 (0.57)

of the more challenging children in the disaffected cluster, who were potentially less likely to do well in foster care, were no longer in foster care at the two-year point and were therefore not included in the analysis.

Generally speaking, then, it appears that foster children make psychosocial gains soon after placement in care, and these early gains tend to be maintained at least up to the two-year point. While these are encouraging results that speak well of foster care, we have not yet heard from the foster children themselves about their experiences. In the next section we report results of two separate studies into children's satisfaction with the care they received.

Children's satisfaction with care

The first of our consumer satisfaction studies focused on short- to medium-term placements and included a sub-set of children from our intake sample who had been in care for approximately six months. Because some of the children who started out in foster care were by then living in CRCs (residential care), children in residential care were also included in this part of the study so that foster care could be compared by children in our sample with its main alternative. The second feedback study assessed the level of satisfaction of children living in stable, long-term foster placements. In order to complete this second study, it was necessary to look beyond the sample included in the tracking study to a supplementary group of children who had been in the one foster home for years.

Children in short- to medium-term care

In the first child satisfaction study, a total of 51 children (23 girls, 28 boys) with a mean age of 11.68 ($SD = 2.82$) were interviewed. Of these, 15 (29.4 per cent) were aged ten years or younger, and 36 (70.6 per cent) were aged eleven to fifteen years. Seven children (14 per cent) were Aboriginal and 44 (86 per cent) were non-Aboriginal children with Anglo-European ethnic backgrounds. Forty-seven (92 per cent) were from metropolitan Adelaide and 4 (8 per cent) were from the regional areas. Twelve of the children were in residential care and 39 were in foster placements at the time of interview. These children were selected, based upon approval and availability, from our larger longitudinal study cohort. As previously indicated, all children were interviewed approximately six months after they entered the study. Permission to interview the children was obtained from social workers, foster carers and, of course, from the children themselves.

The children in the sub-sample had experienced a mean of 7.58 ($SD = 8.16$) previous placements when the longitudinal study began and a mean of 119.90 ($SD = 170.72$) weeks in care. This did not differ significantly from the mean number of placements of children not included in the study ($M = 6.05$,

Table 7.10 Problems experienced by the sub-sample at intake, *n*, (%) (*n* = 51)

Active abuse	
Physical abuse	11 (22)
Sexual abuse	6 (12)
Emotional abuse	17 (33)
Unspecified abuse	4 (8)
Parental problems	
Neglect	16 (31)
Parental incapacity	11 (22)
Child problems	
Child incapacity	13 (25)
Child mental health	8 (16)
Homelessness	7 (14)
Behaviour	30 (59)

$SD = 6.73$), t (229) = 1.36, $p > 0.05$, or from the amount of time previously in care ($M = 76.27$, $SD = 140.88$), t (229) = 1.85, $p > 0.05$. A summary of problems experienced by the children at intake is provided in Table 7.10, which indicates that behavioural problems, neglect and abuse were the most prevalent problems at that point.

Approximately a quarter of the children had significant physical or mental problems (child incapacity). Approximately 25 per cent were in care because their parents were unable to provide care owing to mental illness, substance misuse or incarceration (parental incapacity). These background characteristics of the group were compared with those of children who were not interviewed. No significant differences were found between groups in background characteristics (all $\chi^2 < 1$). There were also no differences in psychosocial adjustment scores (conduct, hyperactivity, emotionality) at any follow-up point, or in the number of placements and amount of time spent in care prior to the reference placement. Taken as a whole, then, the sample interviewed was representative of the children in the larger longitudinal study in terms of background characteristics.

Children in the feedback study were asked a number of questions relating to their satisfaction with their social worker, including whether they knew the name of their FAYS worker, how often they saw that worker (1 = once a week, 2 = at least monthly, 3 = less than once a month), whether their worker listened to them and cared for them (1 = a lot, 2 = a fair bit, 3 = not much, 4 = not at all), and how helpful their worker had been (out of 10, where 1 = really unhelpful and 10 = really helpful). Children were also asked to rate their current placement (yes/no) in terms of whether they felt secure, their carer understood them, showed interest in them, treated them well, and whether the rules and discipline were reasonable. The level of the care received by the children was assessed using Barber and Delfabbro's (2000b) fourteen-item Caregiving Scale. This scale asks respondents to rate how often various actions have been undertaken towards, or with the involvement of, the child by his or her self-selected primary care giver over the last month (1 = not at all, 2 = once or twice, 3 = a few times, 4 = at least once a day). Sample items include: 'had a conversation', 'shared meals', 'helped with homework', 'praised me for something', 'showed affection'. In their study of 375 adolescents from the general Australian population, Barber and Delfabbro found that the scale possessed an acceptable level of internal consistency ($\alpha = 0.70$) for male and female respondents. From a possible range of 14 (no care) to 56 (maximum care), the mean score within the general population was 33.47 ($SD = 6.57$) with no significant difference between male and female ratings. Children were also asked to rate their happiness with the placement out of 10, where 1 = really unhappy and 10 = really happy. Finally, children were asked (using an open-ended question) to indicate what they would most like to see improved or changed to make their placement better.

Forty-eight (94 per cent) of the children knew the name of their social worker. In the remaining three cases, the name of the worker was unknown because a new worker had recently been appointed and had not, at the time of the interview, been in contact with the child. Of the 49 children who provided frequency of contact data, 10 (20 per cent) reported weekly contact, 15 (30 per cent) reported more than weekly contact, and 24 (49 per cent) reported less than weekly contact. When asked to rate the helpfulness of their social worker out of 10, the mean score was 7.74 ($SD = 2.50$), indicating a high level of satisfaction. However, 12 children (23.5 per cent) gave a score of 5 or lower. Ratings did not differ depending upon whether children were in foster care or residential care, t (48) < 1.

Children were also asked whether their social worker cared for and was willing to listen to them. Only 7 (14 per cent) of children said that their worker listened 'not at all' or 'not very much'. Similarly, only 8 (16 per cent) gave a similar score for caring. Over 90 per cent of children believed that their worker both cared for and listened to them. Once again, these satisfaction ratings did not vary according to placement type.

Table 7.11 summarizes children's assessments of their current placement. This table shows that almost all children in foster care were generally very satisfied with the standard of care they received. Fisher Exact tests showed that children in residential care reported feeling significantly less secure and well-treated compared with children in foster care ($p < 0.05$). Children were also asked to rate (out of 10) how happy they were in their present placement. Children were generally very happy ($M = 8.00$, $SD = 2.37$), and this did not differ significantly depending upon whether children were in residential or foster care, t (48) = 2.00, $p > 0.05$.

Table 7.11 Children's assessment of placement, n, (%)

	Foster placements (n = 39)	Residential care (n = 12)	Total sample (n = 51)
Secure	39 (100)	8 (67)	47 (92)
Carer understands you	37 (95)	8 (67)	45 (88)
Carer shows interest	37 (95)	8 (67)	45 (88)
Well treated	39 (100)	8 (67)	47 (92)
Rules and discipline acceptable	36 (92)	8 (67)	44 (86)

A final set of analyses examined satisfaction ratings broken into two age groups: those ten years and younger, and those aged eleven years and older. Mann-Whitney tests revealed no significant differences between groups for ratings of the social worker's willingness to listen, helpfulness or care, nor in the overall rating of happiness. Chi-square tests revealed no significant association between age group and the remaining satisfaction measures scored on binary scales.

Correlation analysis was undertaken to identify the factors associated with satisfaction ratings. (This analysis was confined to foster children because of the likely confounding effect of placement type.) Social workers who were rated as more helpful were also more likely to listen, r (39) = 0.37, $p < 0.05$, and to care for the children, r (39) = 0.50, $p < 0.01$. Satisfaction with social workers was not related to how often the worker was in contact, nor with how satisfied children were with their placements. Children's happiness in placement was also unrelated to the frequency of social worker contact and the general quality of the placement (security, quality of treatment or interest shown by the carer). However, the relationship between perceived strictness (i.e., amount of discipline) of the carer and satisfaction approached significance, r (39) = 0.30, $p < 0.10$. Satisfaction with social workers and placements was not associated with the children's psychological adjustment (conduct, hyperactivity or emotionality). Finally, analysis of the relationship between ratings of placement quality showed that carers who provided reasonable discipline were seen as being more understanding than stricter carers, r (39) = 0.70, $p < 0.001$.

The mean score on the care giving scale for the foster care sample was 37.92 (SD = 8.80) and this was significantly higher than scores obtained in Barber and Delfabbro's (2000b) normative sample of children from the general population, t (413) = 3.87, $p < 0.01$ (see above). Correlation analysis (again confined to foster children) showed that children with higher scores on this scale were significantly happier in their placement, r (39) = 0.44, $p < 0.01$.

Children in long-term care

A total of 48 children (23 girls, 25 boys) with a mean age of 13.1 ($SD = 2.40$) were interviewed for the study on satisfaction with long-term care. Six (12.5 per cent) of the children were aged ten years and younger, and 42 (87.5 per cent) were eleven and older. These children were again selected based upon availability and capacity to answer questions about their well-being. All children were non-Aboriginal and drawn from the metropolitan area of Adelaide or country towns within a 50-km radius of the city. The children had been in their current placement for a mean of 5.1 ($SD = 4.65$) years.

The social workers of children in this study were administered the six-item conduct disorder sub-scale described in Chapter 4, and the children were administered a measure of child satisfaction derived from Stuntzner-Gibson, Koren and DeChillo (1995). This latter measure consisted of eleven items relating to the child's satisfaction with placement, including whether the child liked living with the foster family, was able to get help and have fun, and felt supported. Each item was scored on a three-point scale: 1 = yes, 2 = sort of, 3 = no. The mean item score on the conduct disorder sub-scale did not differ from the scores obtained in the larger longitudinal study (this study: $M = 0.67$, $SD = 0.40$; longitudinal study: $M = 0.69$, $SD = 0.54$).

Table 7.12 shows that most children in long-term foster care were satisfied with almost all aspects of their current placement. Foster homes were described as being highly nurturing, although approximately 20 per cent of children believed that they needed more help than they were currently getting and that they did not always get along with their foster carers. There was no significant relationship between how long children had been in care and their satisfaction on any items.

Table 7.12 Children's satisfaction with long-term placements, *n*, (%) (*n* = 48)

	Yes	Sort of	No
Do you like living with this family?	43 (89.6)	4 (8.3)	1 (2.1)
Do you get the sort of care you would hope for?	47 (97.9)	1 (2.1)	0 (0.0)
Do you get help with things you need help with?	43 (89.6)	5 (10.4)	0 (0.0)
Do you need more help than you get?	3 (6.3)	6 (12.5)	39 (81.3)
Do you feel happy with this family?	47 (97.9)	0 (0.0)	1 (2.1)
Do you feel safe with this family?	47 (97.9)	1 (2.1)	0 (0.0)
Do you have fun with this family?	44 (91.7)	3 (6.3)	1 (2.1)
Do you feel at home with this family?	43 (89.6)	3 (6.3)	1 (2.1)
Do you feel wanted and supported?	45 (93.8)	3 (6.3)	0 (0.0)
Does your foster carer listen to you?	40 (83.3)	8 (16.7)	0 (0.0)
Do you think things could be better between you and your foster carer?	6 (12.5)	11 (22.9)	31 (64.6)

General discussion

Generally speaking, then, our findings suggest that foster care is a positive experience for the majority of children. Psychosocial adjustment, as measured by our standardized instruments, appears to improve in the short term, and the gains made are then maintained at least until the two-year point. Around a quarter of the children who need foster care can be expected to return home within four months, rising to around 40 per cent by the end of two years. Furthermore, the results of both consumer feedback studies suggest that foster children are generally very satisfied with their placements. This applied not only to newly placed children but also to those who had been in care for some time. Specifically, both samples reported being happy in their placements, and feeling safe and well looked after by their foster parents. The first feedback study also showed that most children were satisfied with their social workers, most of whom were rated as very helpful, interested in the child's well-being and willing to listen to the child's concerns. These findings are consistent with recent work by Wilson and Conroy (1999), who also found that children in residential care were less satisfied both with their placements and with their social workers than were foster children. In our study, most complaints from residential children related to limit-setting rather than the quality of care. Examples included being unable to smoke, ride their bikes on the road, form relationships with others in the centre, or stay out later at night. Only three children expressed significant concerns, and these related predominantly to the safety of residential units, in particular having to share accommodation with young offenders.

Our findings are also broadly supportive of the work of Johnson, Yoken and Voss (1995), who interviewed 59 early adolescents using a structured interview approach similar to ours and found that the vast majority of the children in foster care reported being satisfied with their time in care and with the services provided by their social worker. And, on the basis of administrative assessments of 1,100 children in the US state of Illinois, Wilson and Conroy (1999) found that approximately 85 per cent of the children in that study reported feeling loved and safe in their current placement, and were satisfied with their quality of life, as measured by their clothes, living environment, food and level of enjoyment. Three-quarters were satisfied with their social workers, although almost half of the children did report having unmet needs. Like us, Wilson and Conroy found that children in foster care were significantly more satisfied than those in group homes. It is also worth noting that the positive feedback we obtained was unlikely to be merely the result of socially desirable responding or selective sampling. In addition to the fact that the children seemed perfectly willing to express their concerns in our interviews, satisfaction ratings were significantly correlated with scores on Barber and Delfabbro's (2000b) Parent Checklist as one would expect of any valid measure of child satisfaction.

Interestingly, although social workers who were rated as more caring were also perceived as being able to listen and helpful, a good social worker in our study was not necessarily one who was in frequent contact with the foster child. It may be that the nature and quality of contact is more important than frequency, or that placements that are successful require very little social worker intervention. Our results also showed that children's happiness and their satisfaction with the quality of care provided are not necessarily related. Although it is important to acknowledge that the absence of statistical association might be due to the limited variability of responses (most children were happy), there are good reasons why such relationships might not always be expected. Prolonged abuse, disillusionment and frustration at not being able to see siblings or parents are only some of the factors contributing to feelings of unhappiness in foster children, and these factors are likely to persist in the best of placements.

While most of this chapter seems encouraging, our study did find a distressing amount of placement instability in foster care. Understandably, the largest amount of disruption occurred in the first four months of placement, with approximately 40 per cent of the sample changing homes at least once in that period. But at each of the subsequent follow-up points, approximately one in five of the children in care at the start of the study period changed placement at least once over the relevant period. Moreover, Figures 7.1–7.4 clearly show at each follow-up point that large numbers of children who had been unstable in the previous period remained that way in the next, and that children who had previously experienced a period of placement stability needed to move to a new arrangement in the subsequent period. Unquestionably, the most stable placement destination was back home to families of origin, but it needs to be recognized that the children who return home are, by definition, those who come from the best functioning families. In Chapter 10, we will pursue the issue of placement stability more closely and examine the role of individual difference variables in accounting for placement breakdown.

Chapter 8

How important is family contact?

Introduction

A fundamental component of alternative care policy and practice through-out the western world is to ensure that foster children remain in contact with their birth families (see Chapter 1). This principle is enshrined in the departmental guidelines (Family and Youth Services 1999) which assert that 'family contact is a process of maintaining meaningful links between children in care and their families and networks of origin'. Under the guidelines, family contact is deemed to be a right of every child in foster care. The South Australian Children's Protection Act (1993) also expresses this view in Section 4 (2) (b) which states that: 'Serious consideration must be given ... to the desirability of ... preserving and strengthening family relationships between the child, the child's parents and other members of the child's family, whether or not the child is to reside within his or her family' (Osborn 2002). Although a variety of reasons have been advanced in the literature to justify the importance assigned to family contact, three arguments tend to predominate. Firstly, parental visiting helps to maintain long-term attachments between children and their families (Poulin 1992). Secondly, family contact increases the likelihood of children being reunified with their families (Fanshel 1975). Thirdly, parental visiting enhances the psychological well-being of children in care (Cantos, Gries and Slis 1997).

The role of contact as a means of strengthening the bonds between children and their birth families is usually couched in terms of attachment theory, which assumes that healthy development is facilitated throughout the lifespan by the formation of a stable emotional bond with at least one care giver (Barber 2003; Bowlby 1969). For children, the existence of a stable attachment figure provides security and a source of identity, and enhances the child's future capacity for care giving through the mutual exchange of affection. Accordingly, the disruption and separation caused by foster placement is thought to generate feelings of anxiety, abandonment, rejection and fear (Grigsby 1994; Littner 1956). In this light, parental contact is seen as a way of mitigating adverse psychological consequences and of maintaining the child's sense of continuity and identity. Children who are visited by their parents should be less likely to feel that they have been abandoned, will have a better sense of 'who they are', and will be reminded that their families are safe and well (Hess 1988). Such children may be more willing to accept and adjust to their time in foster care in the knowledge that their families still care for them, and will be available to them when circumstances change (Fahlberg 1992).

Although intuitively plausible, evidence supporting this view is relatively sparse. While there is general support for the notion that protracted periods in foster care weaken the relationship between children and their biological families (Fanshel 1979; Fanshel and Shinn 1978; Gillespie, Byrne and Workman 1995; Poulin 1985), links between the frequency of visitation and the quality of the parent–child relationship have been harder to discern. For example, whereas Poulin (1985) found a positive correlation between the degree of attachment with biological parents and the frequency of visiting, the exact opposite effect was observed by Fanshel and Shinn (1978). In this early study, non-visited children actually had a stronger relationship with their families than children who were visited. In response to this inconsistency, Poulin (1992) has suggested that relationships between visitation and attachment may be confounded by age. Since children placed at a younger age tend to have stronger attachments with their foster families, age must be taken into account when analysing the relationship between attachment and family contact.

Another commonly encountered argument in the literature is that children who have more frequent contact with their parents are also more likely to be reunified with their birth families (e.g., Cantos, Gries and Slis 1997; Fanshel 1975; Fanshel and Shinn 1978; Holman 1973; Milner 1987; Weinstein 1960). In Fanshel's (1975) detailed study of this topic, it was found that 86 per cent of children who were frequently and consistently visited went home within a five-year study period compared with only 41 per cent who were infrequently visited throughout this period. Furthermore, those for whom there was a change from low to high frequency visiting had a 53 per cent chance of going home, whereas those who experienced a decrease from high to low levels of visitation had only a 35 per cent chance. Intuitively, it does not seem surprising that this would be so. However, as Cantos, Gries and Slis (1997) point out, a limitation of the argument is that it is not possible to draw a clear causal link between reunification and family contact because the relationship is normally confounded by other factors:

> It could be that those parents who are visiting frequently are better adjusted than those parents who visit less and more likely to have their children returned home. The relationship between visiting and discharge may not be a causal one.

(1997, p. 311)

Thus, the frequency of contact may merely reflect the general status of children and parents, and the quality of the relationship between them. Certainly it is the case that, although analyses have been conducted to identify factors associated with parental contact (e.g., Fanshel 1975), very few studies have examined the relationship between visitation and reunification while controlling for other background characteristics. This increases the suspicion that 'easier' cases, such as those involving parents afflicted by mild or short-term illnesses, are more likely to receive frequent family contact and to have a greater likelihood of reunification than those involving parents with more serious physical, psychological or social problems. In support of this contention, research by Fanshel (1975) has shown that family contact is least likely where children have been abandoned or neglected by their parents, but more likely where parents have less intractable problems such as short-term psychological illnesses.

Most contentious of all is whether family contact enhances the well-being of children in care. Although there are several studies that have purported to show links between contact and child well-being (Fanshel and Shinn 1978; Thorpe 1974), all these studies have based their conclusions on unstandardized measures of behavioural adjustment and have often been overly reliant on anecdotal evidence. An attempt to address this issue was undertaken by Cantos, Gries and Slis (1997), who administered the Child Behaviour Checklist (Achenbach 1991) to foster parents. Consistent with predictions, children who were more frequently visited were less likely to display behaviour problems. Unfortunately, as Cantos, Gries and Slis (1997) concede, the association between contact and adjustment did little to unravel the issue of causality, in that less difficult children may well have been more likely to be visited, rather than being better adjusted because they were visited. Furthermore, Cantos, Gries and Slis's sample included children who were specifically referred for treatment of conduct disorder, and this necessarily limits the extent to which their findings can be generalized to the general foster care population. In fact, when Cantos, Gries and Slis (1997) analysed the relationship between visiting and adjustment in a sample of 19 non-referred children, no significant differences were observed between children who were frequently visited and those who were not visited. Once again, the results seem to suggest that less difficult, better adjusted children are more likely to be visited by their parents.

The case in support of family contact would be greatly strengthened if it could be shown that: (1) increases in family contact are associated with increases in child well-being and better family relationships, or (2) changes in family contact are associated with changes in the likelihood of reunification. So far neither proposition has been conclusively proved. Instead, the impression given by some researchers is that family contact can actually place considerable emotional strain on children by reminding them of the separation (Pithouse and Parry 1997); it can generate a conflict of loyalties between biological and foster parents (Simms and Bolden 1991); it can increase social worker workloads (Cleaver 1997), and increase conflicts between parents and children (Cleaver 1997). Indeed, some have argued that contact arrangements often have more to do with satisfying law courts than with the best interests of the child (Cleaver 1998; Hess 1988; Gillespie, Byrne and Workman 1995).

The purpose of the present chapter, then, is to examine the role of family contact over time. More specifically, we examine changes in the extent and nature of family contact in foster care; the correlates of family contact; and the perceived relationship between family contact and family relationships. We also examine whether family contact is related to scores on standardized measures of child adjustment or to the likelihood of reunification.

Family contact after four and eight months in care

As described in Chapter 4, social workers were asked to rate how often the children had been in contact with their birth parents during the previous four months. Three types of contact were considered: (1) indirect or tele-phone contact, (2) direct visits or contact, which referred to physical visits or contacts with the parents without any overnight stays, and (3) overnight stays. The frequency of each form of contact was measured on six-point scales: 1 = never, 2 = monthly or less often, 3 = 2–3 times a month, 4 = once a week, 5 = 2–6 times a week, and 7 = daily or more often. Social workers had no difficulty providing details of visits and overnight stays, since these records are routinely maintained by FAYS' workers. Although no specific records were maintained for telephone contacts between children and their families, workers were confident of their category estimates. Most social workers (70 per cent) were in at least weekly contact with foster carers, and 23 per cent were in contact with carers on at least a monthly basis. Social workers were also asked to rate whether the contact between the child and their families had been beneficial, where 1 = not beneficial, 2 = somewhat beneficial, 3 = very beneficial. They were also asked to rate whether there had been any improvement in the relationship between the children and their families in the period since the last assessment (four months): 1 = very much improved, 2 = slightly improved, 3 = unchanged, 4 = slightly deterior-ated, 5 = very much deteriorated. Finally, they were asked to rate whether the probability of the child being reunified with their families had increased or decreased since the previous assessment point.

Table 8.1 summarizes the number and percentage of children receiving each type of contact during the first and second follow-up periods, including only those cases where data were available at both points in time. The results show that approximately 25 per cent of children were having no contact with their parents by the end of the second (eight-month) follow-up period, approximately 50 per cent were in direct contact and approximately

Table 8.1 Nature of contact during the first and second follow-up periods, n, (%) (n = 132)

	4 months	8 months
No contact	26 (19.7)	32 (24.2)
Indirect or telephone contact	66 (50.0)	61 (46.2)
Direct visits or contact	79 (59.8)	65 (49.2)
Overnight stays	26 (19.7)	24 (18.2)

Table 8.2 Frequency distribution of contact in the first two follow-up periods, n, (%) (note: percentages are based on row totals)

	Once a month or less	2–3 times a month	Once a week	Twice or more a week
Indirect or telephone contact				
First follow-up (n = 66)	13 (19.7)	12 (18.2)	25 (37.9)	16 (24.2)
Second follow-up (n = 61)	16 (26.2)	10 (16.4)	25 (41.0)	8 (13.1)
Direct contact or visits				
First follow-up (n = 79)	25 (31.6)	19 (24.1)	22 (27.8)	6 (7.5)
Second follow-up (n = 66)	12 (18.5)	20 (30.8)	22 (33.8)	12 (18.5)
Overnight stays				
First follow-up (n = 26)	9 (34.6)	10 (38.5)	4 (15.4)	1 (3.8)
Second follow-up (n = 27)	11 (45.8)	8 (33.3)	5 (20.8)	3 (12.5)

Note
Owing to some missing data items on the frequency of contact, not all figures sum to the row totals.

25 per cent were allowed overnight stays. McNemar change tests revealed a significant decrease in the percentage of children having direct contact between the first and second follow-up periods, $\chi^2(1) = 4.23$, $p < 0.05$.

The same tests applied to the frequency of contact data (collapsed into two categories for each time period: once a week or more versus less than once a week) showed that the frequency of each type of contact had not changed across the two time periods (Table 8.2).

Reunification, family relationships and psychological functioning

As expected, statistical analysis showed a significant association between reunification and family contact in the first four months (the period during which most children are reunified – see also Chapter 7). Of the 59 children who were reunified within the four-month period, only 7 had not been in contact with their parents. Children who had telephone or indirect contact

Table 8.3 Social worker assessment of the effects of family contact, n, (%)

Has contact been beneficial? (*n* = 90)

	Not at all beneficial	Somewhat beneficial	Very beneficial
First follow-up	14 (15.6)	56 (62.2)	20 (22.2)
Second follow-up	15 (16.7)	49 (54.4)	23 (25.6)

Nature of relationship between child and birth family (*n* = 92)

	Much improved	Slightly improved	No change	Slightly worse	Much worse
First follow-up	9 (9.8)	24 (26.1)	44 (47.8)	11 (12.0)	4 (4.3)
Second follow-up	7 (7.6)	13 (14.1)	55 (59.8)	11 (12.0)	6 (6.5)

Likelihood of reunification (*n* = 90)

	Increased	Decreased	No change
First follow-up	17 (18.9)	9 (10.0)	64 (71.1)
Second follow-up	10 (11.1)	14 (15.6)	65 (72.2)

(the most frequent form of contact recorded) were significantly more likely to be reunified than those who had no telephone contact (41 out of 52 = 79 per cent for reunified children versus 88 out of 176 = 50 per cent for those who were not reunified), $\chi^2(1) = 13.60$, $p < 0.001$. A Wilcoxon-rank-sum test showed that telephone contact also occurred significantly more frequently for children who went on to be reunified with their parents (mean rank = 142.7 versus 105.21 for non-reunified children), $z = 3.76$, $p < 0.001$.

As indicated in Chapter 4, social workers were also asked to rate the perceived effects of family contact within each follow-up period. The ratings included assessments of how beneficial the contacts had been, whether there had been any improvement or deterioration in the relationship between the child and his or her birth family, and whether there had been any increase or decrease in likelihood of reunification. Only those children who were receiving family contact during both follow-up periods were included in the analysis (Table 8.3). The results in Table 8.3 provide a general description of how family contacts and child–family relationships were perceived in the two follow-up periods. Table 8.3 shows that the majority of social workers perceived contact favourably, with 80 per cent believing that it was 'somewhat' or 'very' beneficial for the child. At the same time, most social workers (60 per cent) did not perceive any change in the relationship between children and their families, or in the likelihood that the child would be

Table 8.4 Perceived effect of changes in the frequency of contact upon the relationship between children and birth families, n, (%)

	Relationship improved	No change	Deteriorated
Indirect or telephone contact			
No change (n = 78)	7 (8.9)	57 (73)	14 (17.9)
Increased (n = 21)	10 (47.6)	9 (42.9)	2 (9.5)
Decreased (n = 33)	9 (27.3)	12 (36.4)	12 (36.4)
Direct visits or contact			
No change (n = 63)	9 (14.3)	39 (61.9)	15 (23.8)
Increased (n = 33)	10 (30.3)	16 (48.5)	7 (21.2)
Decreased (n = 36)	7 (19.4)	23 (63.9)	6 (16.7)
Overnight stays			
No change (n = 96)	15 (15.6)	62 (64.6)	19 (19.8)
Increased (n = 21)	9 (42.9)	8 (38.1)	4 (19.0)
Decreased (n = 15)	2 (13.3)	8 (53.3)	5 (33.3)

reunified (72 per cent). Moreover, approximately 15 to 20 per cent believed that family contact was not beneficial and that the relationship between visited children and their parents had actually deteriorated over time.

A further analysis examined how changes in the frequency of each type of family contact across the two follow-up periods influenced family relationships, including for all children whether or not they had been in contact with their parents. Considering each type of contact separately, this analysis was conducted using three groups: those children who had experienced an increase in contact, those who had experienced a decrease in contact and those for whom there had been no change (Table 8.4). Chi-square tests revealed significant associations between group membership and ratings (all $p < 0.001$) for all three types of contact. Firstly, where there was 'no change' in frequency of family contact, there was also, not surprisingly, 'no change' in the status of the relationship between children and birth families. Secondly, although improvements in relationships tended to coincide with increases in contact (and vice versa for deteriorations), these trends were not statistically significant.

Results for psychological measures were consistent with those for family relationships. Difference scores for measures of psychological adjustment were calculated by subtracting adjustment scores at the end of the second follow-up period from those obtained at the end of the first. These difference scores were compared across the three groups identified above to determine whether changes in the frequency of family contact were associated with corresponding changes in psychological adjustment. No significant group differences were observed, all $F^s < 1$.

Predictors of family contact at eight months

Univariate analyses were undertaken to identify factors associated with each type of family contact (indirect, direct and overnight stays) up to the end of the second follow-up period. Variables found to be significantly associated with each type of contact were then analysed using logistic regression with contact (0 = not occurred, 1 = occurred) as the binary dependent variable for each of the three analyses. Potential predictors considered included: gender, age, ethnicity, metropolitan versus rural, baseline psychological adjustment measures, reasons for being in care and the number of previous placements experienced prior to entering our study. Furthermore, in the light of previous research by Fanshel and Shinn (1978) which has shown that family contact is associated with the length of time children are in care, separate analyses were undertaken using two sub-groups: (1) those children who had entered care for the first time when the study commenced, and (2) those who were already in care and were merely changing to a new placement when the study commenced. (The group 'coming into care' consisted of children who had never been in care before and also those who had been in care some time earlier, but had been home when they were referred for a new placement (the reference placement) that brought them into the study.)

For the overall sample, indirect or telephone contact was more likely to occur for metropolitan than for rural children (54 out of 105 = 51 per cent versus 11 out of 40 = 28 per cent), $\chi^2(1) = 6.71$, $p < 0.01$. Non-Aboriginal children were more likely to have direct contact compared with Aboriginal children (65 out of 122 = 53 per cent versus 4 out of 23 = 17 per cent), $\chi^2(1) = 9.99$, $p < 0.01$. Children who received direct contact were also significantly less likely to be hyperactive at intake ($M = 1.02$, $SD = 0.67$ versus $M = 1.30$, $SD = 0.63$), $t(132) = 2.50$, $p < 0.05$, and had also spent less time (in weeks) in care prior to the reference placement ($M = 86.56$, $SD = 166.27$ versus $M = 155.55$, $SD = 203.73$), $t(140) = 2.22$, $p < 0.05$. Children who were allowed overnight stays had also spent less time in foster care ($M = 71.24$, $SD = 125.08$ versus $M = 136.89$, $SD = 201.35$), $t(140) = 2.19$, $p < 0.05$. Logistic regression was undertaken in two ways to test the stability of the final model: (1) a standard sequential ('Enter') analysis using the Wald statistic, and (2) a stepwise (backwards elimination) analysis with the log-linear likelihood ratio as the test statistic. Both methods produced the same set of significant predictors (parameters, for the latter analysis), so the standard analysis using the Wald statistic will be presented. As indicated in Table 8.5, metropolitan children were over three times (1/0.33) more likely to receive indirect contact than rural children were. Direct contact was more than three and a half times (1/0.28) more likely for non-Aboriginal children, around half as likely for children with hyperactivity (1/0.49), and also less likely the longer children had previously spent in foster care.

Table 8.5 Logistic regression analysis of predictors of family contact during the second (8-month) follow-up period

	Coefficient	Wald	Odds-ratio
Total sample			
Indirect/telephone contact			
Metropolitan–rural	−1.10	7.04**	0.33
Direct visits or contact			
Aboriginality	−1.27	4.32*	0.28
Time in care	< −0.01	4.54*	< 1.00
Hyperactivity	−0.72	6.10*	0.49
Children entering care			
Indirect contact			
Hyperactivity	−1.44	8.68**	0.24
Children already in care			
Indirect contact			
Metropolitan–rural	−1.86	9.56**	0.15
Direct contact			
Time in care	< −0.01†	7.27**	< 1.00
Overnight stays			
Emotional abuse	1.85	8.21**	6.36

Note
* $p < 0.05$ ** $p < 0.01$
Coefficients are very small because of the relatively small effect of one-unit (one-week) increments in the 'time in care' variable.

Chi-square analyses restricted to children who had entered foster care for the first time showed that Aboriginal children were significantly less likely to receive direct contact from their birth families compared with non-Aboriginal children (0 out of 11 = 0 per cent versus 32 out of 50 = 64 per cent), $\chi^2 (1) = 14.81$, $p < 0.001$. Rural children were less likely to receive direct contact compared with metropolitan children (3 out of 12 = 25 per cent versus 29 out of 49 = 59 per cent), $\chi^2 (1) = 6.71$, $p < 0.01$. Children who were in direct contact with their families also scored significantly lower on measures of conduct disorder ($M = 0.53$, $SD = 0.53$ versus $M = 0.86$, $SD = 0.51$), $t (50) = 2.30$, $p < 0.05$, and hyperactivity ($M = 0.80$, $SD = 0.75$ versus $M = 1.46$, $SD = 0.53$), $t (50) = 3.69$, $p < 0.001$ at intake into care. Logistic regression analysis conducted using these variables (Table 8.5) and direct contact as the dependent measure showed that only hyperactivity remained significant when other variables were controlled. Specifically, each unit increase in hyperactivity scores was associated with a 4.17 times decreased likelihood of direct contact.

Chi-square analysis restricted to children who had a prior history of foster care showed that metropolitan children were significantly more likely to receive indirect contact from their parents (29 out of 56 = 52 per cent versus 4 out of 28 = 14 per cent), $\chi^2(1) = 11.01$, $p < 0.001$. Children who were in care because of emotional abuse were more likely to have overnight stays (7 out of 18 = 39 per cent versus 6 out of 66 = 9 per cent), $\chi^2(1) = 9.60$, $p < 0.01$. Finally, children who had direct contact with their parents had spent significantly less time (weeks) in care before entering the study ($M = 121.67$, $SD = 137.17$ versus $M = 243.53$, $SD = 215.75$), $t(50) = 3.13$, $p < 0.01$. Logistic regression (Table 8.5) showed that metropolitan children were $(1/0.15) = 6.67$ times more likely to receive indirect contact. Each week previously in placement led to a reduction in the likelihood of direct contact, whereas children who were in care because of emotional abuse were 6.36 times more likely to stay overnight.

Family contact after one year in care

Of the 128 children still in care at twelve months, 33 (25.7 per cent) had no contact with their families, 54 (42.2 per cent) had indirect contact, 69 (53.9 per cent) had direct contact and 16 (12.5 per cent) had overnight stays. These figures do not differ significantly from those obtained at the eight-month point (see Table 8.1). Of the 91 cases for whom the relevant data were available, there were 12 cases (13.2 per cent) where social workers felt that the contact was not beneficial, 49 (53.8 per cent) that were indifferent and 30 (32.9 per cent) where the contact was thought to be beneficial. Thus, social workers' views about contact arrangements at twelve months were mixed, although somehat more positive than negative.

Reunification, family relationships and psychological functioning

The first aim of the analyses reported in this section was to ascertain whether variations in the frequency of contact between four months (the earliest available point) and one year had influenced placement outcomes, family relationships or psychosocial adjustment. As previously indicated, this study included both objective and subjective measures of reunification. The objective measure was simply the number of children who went home to their birth families and stayed there throughout the study period, and the subjective measure asked social workers to estimate the likelihood of reunification at the end of the relevant follow-up period. This was measured on a three-point scale, where 1 = increased likelihood, 2 = decreased likelihood and 3 = no change. Although this subjective measure could be questioned on the grounds that the decision to reunify is not the social worker's alone, recent research conducted by the Department of Family and Youth Services in

South Australia has shown that children rarely go home if their social worker has no 'intention to reunify' (Forward and Carver 1999). Thus, the views of social workers are clearly critical in the reunification process.

Objective analysis showed that the vast majority of children who went home in the first year of care did so in the first four months (see also Chapter 7). Because only 4 children went home in the eight- to twelve-month period, it is not possible to consider how changes in family contact across twelve months affected actual reunification rates. However, it was possible to cross-tabulate the three contact groups identified above (direct, indirect, overnight stays) with the social workers' optimism concerning reunification at the end of twelve months. Overall, 80 (77 per cent) social workers (valid cases = 104) said that there had been no change in the likelihood of reunification, 15 (14 per cent) said that there was a decreased likelihood and 9 (8 per cent) said that there was an increased likelihood. Further analyses revealed no significant association between changes in each type of contact and social worker estimates of the likelihood of reunification. In other words, children for whom there had been a change in frequency of contact were not seen by social workers as having any changed likelihood of returning home.

In order to examine the effects of longer-term variations in contact upon family relationships, three groups were constructed for each contact type, where 1 = no change in the frequency of contact, 2 = increase in frequency of contact, 3 = decrease. These were validated by conducting separate within-group comparisons for the 'increase' and 'decrease' groups to confirm that each had experienced a statistically significant change in contact from the four-month to the twelve-month assessment point. Overall, t-tests confirmed that groups classified as having an increase or decrease in contact had experienced significant increases or decreases in contact in the period specified ($p < 0.001$). Next, social workers' ratings of changes in the relationship between children and their birth families were examined in relation to the changes in contact that had occurred throughout the year. Table 8.6 summarizes the quality of the relationship between the child and his or her birth family at the end of twelve months, and the status of family contacts across

Table 8.6 Mean, (SD) of family strain in relation to contact variations, 4–12 months (higher scores indicate a poorer relationship)

	No change	Increased	Decreased
Telephone contact	2.79 (0.83) (n = 43)	2.73 (1.01) (n = 30)	3.17 (0.89) (n = 35)
Direct contact	2.90 (0.80) (n = 41)	2.63 (0.92) (n = 41)	3.23 (0.99) (n = 26)
Overnight stays	2.83 (0.90) (n = 78)	2.33 (0.89) (n = 12)	3.44 (0.70) (n = 18)

the twelve-month period. One-way ANOVA applied to indirect contact data revealed no significant difference across the three groups, $F (2, 105) = 2.40$, $p > 0.05$. There was, however, a significant difference for direct contact, $F (2, 105) = 3.57$, $p < 0.05$. Fisher post-hoc tests showed that the children who experienced a decrease in direct contact were more likely to display a deteriorating relationship with their birth families at the twelve-month point ($p < 0.05$). There was also a significant group difference for overnight stays, $F (2, 105) = 6.23$, $p < 0.01$, with post-hoc comparisons showing that the group which had experienced a decrease in contact had a significantly poorer relationship with their birth family than the other two groups had ($p < 0.05$). The effect sizes for these comparisons were all large and ranged from 0.63 to 1.42.

Finally, Pearson correlation analysis was used to examine changes in psychosocial adjustment (four to twelve months) in relation to variations in the frequency of each type of contact. No significant correlation was obtained.

Predictors of family contact at one year

Univariate analyses similar to those employed at eight months were applied to the twelve-month data. These revealed only one significant finding: Aboriginal children were significantly less likely to have any form of contact with their birth families compared with non-Aboriginal children. This relationship was obtained for the overall sample and was evident also when the analysis was further broken down into those who were already in care and those who had entered care for the first time when the study commenced. Whereas only 6 out of 20 (30 per cent) Aboriginal children in the overall sample had any direct contact with their parents, for example, 63 out of 107 (58.9 per cent) of the non-Aboriginal children in the sample had direct contact.

Family contact after two years in care

Of the 103 children for whom there was valid data at the two-year point, 25 (22.9 per cent) had no family contact; 33 (32.0 per cent) had telephone contact; 56 (54.3 per cent) had direct visits, and 16 (15.5 per cent) had overnight stays. Again, these percentages did not significantly differ from the figures obtained at early assessment points. The principal focus of the analyses presented in this section was to examine the effects of contact based upon the earliest (four months) and latest data (two years) that were available. The first issue investigated was whether there was any evidence to support Fanshel's (1975) contention that the frequency of family contact decreases the longer children remain in care. This was investigated by comparing the earliest available contact data (four months) with the data for children remaining in care at the two-year point. This involved a comparison of the estimated average number of visits a year received by the child at each point in time. Of the total of 58 cases with valid data available at both points, 11 (19.0 per cent) had the same rate of contact at two years; 33 had an increased rate of contact (56.9 per cent); and 12 (20.7 per cent) had a decreased rate of contact. A chi-square goodness of fit test confirmed that, contrary to established wisdom, children in this study were significantly more likely to experience an increase in the frequency of direct contact rather than a decrease from four months to two years, $\chi^2(1) = 9.8$, $p < 0.001$. A t-test comparison of the absolute frequency of contact revealed that the rate was significantly higher at two years ($M = 62.41$, $SD = 72.5$) than at four months ($M = 28.41$, $SD = 46.4$), $t(57) = 3.20$, $p < 0.01$ (effect size = 0.58).

Before this result is taken at face value, however, it is important to recognize that the analysis was not based solely upon children coming into care for the first time, so that any relationship between time in care and change in family contact could be oversimplified in that it ignores a child's previous placement history. Thus, any family contact changes for the group already in care refer to a potentially longer period in care than two years. In order to assess whether the changes applied to both groups, then, t-test comparisons were repeated for each group separately. These showed that the effect was indeed replicated across both groups, but even more strongly in the group already in care. For the group already in care ($M = 19.65$, $SD = 36.2$ versus $M = 49.2$, $SD = 60.9$), $t(33) = 3.18$, $p < 0.01$ (effect size = 0.55), and for the group entering care for the first time ($M = 40.83$, $SD = 56.4$ versus $M = 80.1$, $SD = 84.1$), $t(23) = 1.81$, $p = 0.08$ (effect size = 0.40).

Reunification, family relationships and psychological functioning

When asked to indicate the likelihood of children being reunified with their parents at two years, only 2 (3.7 per cent) of the 54 workers who answered this question indicated that there had been any change. Despite this, social workers remained positive about the role of family contact. Of 72 cases with valid data, 62 (86.1 per cent) rated the contact as beneficial, and only 10 (14.0 per cent) rated it as unhelpful. Quality of family relationship scores were compared across three groups: those who experienced an increase in contact, no change in contact, and those with a decrease in contact. A one-way ANOVA revealed no significant difference in scores, $F(2, 55) = 1.42$, $p > 0.05$, indicating that variations in contact frequency from four to twelve months did not influence longer-term family functioning scores. There was also no correlation between changes in family functioning ratings (four months to two years) and changes in frequency of direct contact. A final analysis examined variations in psychological adjustment (four months to two years) in relation to variations in the frequency of contact (four months to two years). This revealed no significant correlation between change in visiting and change in adjustment.

Predictors of family contact at two years

Once again, a series of univariate analyses was undertaken to identify the factors that were associated with family contact after two years. Encouragingly, the association between Aboriginality and a lower rate of contact was no longer significant at two years. The results for this analysis varied considerably depending upon whether children had entered care for the first time or were merely changing placements when the study began. For those children who came into care, direct contact was significantly more likely if the placement had arisen as a result of parental incapacity (12 out of 15 = 80 per cent incapacity versus 10 out of 23 = 43.5 per cent no incapacity), $\chi^2(1) = 4.97, p < 0.05$. The most striking finding for this group of children, however, was that those with direct family contact had significantly poorer psychosocial functioning scores at the two-year point: conduct ($M = 0.65$, $SD = 0.56$ versus $M = 0.28$, $SD = 0.31$ for no contact), $t(36) = 2.40, p < 0.05$; hyperactivity ($M = 1.20$, $SD = 0.62$ versus $M = 0.64$, $SD = 0.58$ for no contact), $t(36) = 2.83, p < 0.01$; emotionality ($M = 0.91$, $SD = 0.60$ versus $M = 0.54$, $SD = 0.38$ for no contact), $t(36) = 2.20, p < 0.05$. The effect sizes for these differences were all very large (0.90+). By contrast, for those already in care when the study began, there was a significant association between gender and direct contact, with a greater proportion of boys (37 out of 58 = 63.8 per cent) than girls (19 out of 44 = 43.2 per cent) having direct contact, $\chi^2(1) = 4.29, p < 0.05$ at two years.

General discussion

The results presented in this chapter are not altogether straightforward, but it is none the less possible to draw out a number of general conclusions about the role of family contact in foster care. The most important of these are as follows:

*   There is little evidence to suggest that children who remain in care for longer periods necessarily experience a gradual decrease in the frequency of family contact.
*   Children who are in frequent contact with their parents in the early months of foster care tend to have a higher probability of being reunified with their families.
*   Social workers also generally believe that family contact is beneficial for children.
*   In the longer term, there is little apparent relationship between changes in the frequency of contact and the likelihood of reunification.
*   Although family contact and reunification are correlated, they do not appear to be causally linked.

- In the early months after intake, children with poorer behavioural adjustment at intake are less likely to be visited, but the reverse is so for children who are in care for two years.
- Aboriginal children are less likely to have contact with their birth families, particularly in the first few months after being placed into care.

In short, our results are consistent with some aspects of foster care practice wisdom and inconsistent with others. Consistent with Fanshel and Shinn's (1978) detailed study of the topic, for example, family contact was found to be positively associated with reunification and was also less frequent for minority children. Furthermore, we have confirmed previous research showing that more difficult (in our case, more hyperactive) children are less likely to have parental contact. On the other hand, while there was some evidence of a decrease in direct family contact in the months following intake, there was no convincing evidence to support Fanshel and Shinn's (1978) view that children tend to lose touch with their parents the longer they spend in care. Surprisingly, our results showed precisely the opposite. A possible reason for the discrepancy is that, whereas we tracked family contact among the same children over time, Fanshel and Shinn took repeated cross-sectional measures. This meant that the children in Fanshel and Shinn's study at the end were a qualitatively different sample of children from those who began, so the apparent decline in family contact that they observed could have been a result of selection bias.

Another difference between our findings and conventional practice wisdom relates to the notion that family contact enhances short-term reunification and helps to enhance family connections. Although these statistical associations were replicated within our sample, at least in the short term, there was no evidence that change in family contact influenced likelihood of reunification over the longer term. It therefore seems likely that the relationship between contact and reunification is correlational rather than causal. In this sense, our results suggest a somewhat more mundane conclusion than is common in the foster care literature: simply that children who get along well with their families, and who are in care as a result of less serious problems, tend to have more frequent contact with their parents and are likely to go home sooner. The results in this chapter also suggest that the relationship between family contact and the child's psychosocial adjustment is more complex than has been suggested by previous literature. Although, as might be expected, there was a negative association between psychosocial adjustment and contact in the early months (less well-adjusted children tended to have less contact), this relationship was reversed after two years. At two years, those children who were in direct contact with their birth parents displayed significantly *poorer* psychological adjustment. Why this should be so is not immediately obvious; however, the fact that this association was obtained only for those children coming into care for the first time may suggest that a point is eventually reached where family contact becomes distressing for children who have not previously been separated from their parents for long periods. Alternatively, it may be that the connection between family contact and psychological distress is explained by emotional closeness between child and family of origin. In other words, children who are closer to their families are more likely both to be visited and to be more distressed by protracted separation.

As Hess and Proch (1988) point out, courts very often insist on contact between parents and children on the assumption that this is in the best interests of the child. An adverse consequence of this may be that it serves to intensify children's sense of loss if the separation continues and may undermine foster carers' attempts to build a relationship with the child in their care. Indeed, just this view has been expressed by Adcock (1980), who has argued for clearer justification of parental access on the grounds that parental visiting can 'create anxiety which is detrimental to their children's security' especially when 'many parents who visit have not accepted they cannot have their children back' (p. 24). Similarly, Gean, Gillmore and Dowler (1985) have argued that visiting can involve considerable stress for all parties – the foster child, the biological parents and the foster parents. These authors stated that foster children often feel a conflict of loyalties between the biological parents and their foster parents, and react in an angry and confused manner during and after visits. This phenomenon has also been reported by Schofield, Beek and Sargent (2000), who found that at least a third of foster children experienced stress and potential harm as a result of interacting with parents and grandparents during their time in care.

Chapter 9

The predictors of family reunification

Introduction

In the previous chapter, we reported that there was little evidence to support a causal connection between family contact and family reunification. This finding raises the vital question: what does enhance the likelihood of reunification? As discussed in Chapter 1, child protection jurisdictions throughout the world continue to place a very high priority on returning foster children to their families of origin as soon as possible wherever feasible. It is therefore expected that a significant proportion of worker time and resources will be directed towards the implementation of service plans to facilitate reunification. For this reason, identifying which children are most likely to go home and the factors that contribute to reunification have become a central focus of social work research (Courtney 1994; Fanshel and Shinn 1978). By understanding the differential probability of reunification in alternative care samples, it may be possible to target time and resources better. Although the issue of reunification has been subject to investigation for many years, research findings have been many and varied, making it difficult to form a consistent view of what factors enhance reunification success. Nevertheless, several general conclusions can be reached. Firstly, reunification appears to be much more probable in the short term than in the long term. In other words, the chance of reunification decreases the longer children remain in care (Fanshel 1975; Fernandez 1999). Secondly, children who are in regular contact with their families while in care are more likely to go home (see Chapter 8; Bullock, Little and Millham 1993; Farmer and Parker 1991). A third factor is the nature and quality of support provided by the alternative care system. Specifically, reunification is much more likely when there are consistent interactions between birth families and social workers (Berry 1992; Schuerman, Rzepnecki and Johnson 1994), when there are well-established case-management procedures (Turner 1984), when planned services are completed by birth families (Lewis, Walton and Fraser 1995; Nugent, Carpenter and Parks 1993) and when the problems leading to children entering care are more amenable to change. For example, Courtney

(1994) and Benedict and White (1991) found that children with health problems and disabilities were less likely to be reunified. Children who have been sexually abused are generally more likely to go home than are neglected children (Courtney 1994; Farmer 1992); minority children are less likely to be reunified than European children (Benedict and White 1991; Jenkins and Diamond 1985; Seaberg and Tolley 1986); and older children with behavioural problems are less likely to be reunified than children whose parents have illnesses or other incapacities (Fanshel and Shinn 1978).

Despite consistent findings such as these, one of the major difficulties with many studies of reunification is that they fail to take account of a number of conceptual and methodological complexities. These complexities include the need to differentiate between types of reunification, the effect of variations in time frame in statistical analyses, and also the sensitivity of results to variations in sample characteristics (Fernandez 1999). The expression 'reunification type' refers to the fact that reunification can be conceptualized as either a passive or an active process. Passive reunification refers to cases in which children go home without social work intervention because of changes in circumstances and factors largely outside the worker's control. Examples of the external factors leading to reunification include improvements in parental health, the release of parents from prison or the departure of perpetrators in child protection cases (Farmer 1992). Such factors contrast with the active process of reunification brought about by services or interventions set in place by social workers and others in the alternative care system. Examples of factors requiring social work intervention include poor parenting skills, behaviour management problems and ongoing parent–child conflict. Although a neat distinction between external and service-related factors cannot always be made, recognition of the difference is nevertheless vital for identifying the role of services on reunification rates. In order to understand what practices work at what point in time, it is important to be able to exclude those cases where the factors contributing to placement are either transitory or beyond the worker's control from the outset.

The issue of time comes into play here because the characteristics that predict reunification are likely to vary according to the interval that has elapsed since the child's entry into care. For example, Bullock, Little and Millham (1993) found it necessary to distinguish between 'early', 'intermediate' and 'long-term' returners because different predictors were obtained for each group. In addition, results may vary merely because of variations in sample selection across time. Although some studies include only children new to care (e.g., Benedict and White 1991; Courtney 1994; Fernandez 1999), others have included children with pre-existing placement histories (Fanshel, Finch and Grundy 1989). There also may be variations in the length of the reference placement used as the basis for including children in follow-up samples. For example, in some studies a minimum of two weeks in care has been used (e.g., Fernandez 1999), whereas in others (e.g., Fanshel and Shinn 1978) the interval has been several months. As it is highly likely that all three of these factors (type, time and length of reference placement) are interrelated, it may be difficult to make comparisons between different studies. For example, passive reunification may be more likely to occur soon after placement, so that, if one study excludes placements of only a few weeks while another does not, different statistical associations are likely to emerge. Furthermore, significant doubts can be raised about analyses based on the amount of contact between social workers and families, and on the amount of social work that has been devoted to cases (Forward and Carver 1999), because challenging cases (the children who are most difficult to reunify) often attract a greater proportion of social work intervention. Thus, it is conceivable that the likelihood of reunification is inversely related to the amount of work undertaken or the number of interventions implemented. For this reason, it may be difficult to determine the nature of the relationship between service interventions and the likelihood of reunification, unless one confines this analysis to a group of cases that share similar characteristics.

In this chapter, we describe findings from a series of analyses in which we investigated the nature and predictors of family reunification within our sample. In the final section of the chapter, we consider the implications of this work for social work practice.

Predictors of family reunification in the short term

The first analysis that is presented relates to the first four months of foster care. This period is targeted for two reasons: firstly, because this period appears to be the critical time during which the majority of reunifications occur (Fernandez 1999), and, secondly, because the variables thought to predict reunification in this period have been shown to differ from those that lead to reunification when children have been in care for longer periods (Bullock, Little and Millham 1993). In this part of the study, statistical analyses are followed by profile analysis of reunified children to determine what precise changes, factors, or interventions led to reunification. In this way, a more detailed understanding can be obtained of the role and significance of general case characteristics, and of whether this role is consistent across cases with similar characteristics.

Analytical approach

A limitation of some previous analyses (e.g., Fernandez 1999) is that any return home is deemed to constitute reunification. But not all children who return home necessarily stay there. On some occasions, children are sent home for short periods because no other placement option is immediately available; in such cases, there is no intention for children to stay at home. In the analyses that follow, then, only 'complete reunifications' (in which children went home and stayed there until the end of the four-month follow-up period) have been included. Furthermore, in recognition of the fact that this study includes both (1) children changing placements after the break-down of an existing placement ($n = 105$) and (2) those coming into the care system for the first time ($n = 129$), aggregate analyses are followed by additional analyses that test the validity of overall findings for the two groups separately. A total of 49 children were reunified with birth families at the end of the first 120-day follow-up period. Of these children, 41 were from the 'entering care' group, and 8 were in the 'already in care' group.

The data were analysed in two stages. The first stage involved identification of univariate associations between key study variables (described above) and reunification (0 = occurred, 1 = not occurred). In the second stage, all significant univariate predictors were entered into a proportional hazards analysis or Cox regression. This technique has been commonly used in alternative care research and is recommended as the most effective way to analyse reunification data (Benedict and White 1991; Courtney 1994; Fernandez 1999; Goerge 1990). With this technique, the effect of multiple variables on the probability of reunification can be assessed and the probability of reunification expressed as a continuous function of time. This allows a distinction to be drawn between reunifications in general and those that occurred after t days. That is, as well as obtaining the probability of reunification at the end of period P (given certain values on the significant covariates), the probability at $P\text{-}t$ days can also be determined.

Total sample analysis

Using the total sample ($n = 235$), it was found that reunification was significantly less likely for children living in rural areas (6 out of 56 = 11 per cent in rural areas versus 48 out of 179 = 27 per cent in the metropolitan area), $\chi^2 (1) = 6.25$, $p < 0.05$, for Aboriginal children (2 out of 38 = 5 per cent Aboriginal versus 52 out of 197 = 26 per cent non-Aboriginal), $\chi^2 (1) = 8.04$, $p < 0.01$, and for those who were victims of neglect (7 out of 66 = 11 per cent neglect versus 46 out of 168 = 27 per cent other reasons), $\chi^2 (1) = 7.61$, $p < 0.01$. However, reunification was significantly more likely for children whose parents had some form of incapacity, such as physical or mental illness (26 out of 76 = 34 per cent parental incapacity versus 28 out of 159 = 18 per cent no incapacity), $\chi^2 (1) = 8.01$, $p < 0.01$. To understand why these variables might have been associated with reunification, further analyses examined the relationship between these predictors and other key variables. Specifically, neglected children were found to be significantly younger than non-neglected children ($M = 9.68$, $SD = 3.24$ versus $M = 11.20$, $SD = 3.42$), $t (232) = 3.10$, $p < 0.01$, and were also less likely to have behavioural problems (29 out of 66 = 44 per cent with behavioural problems versus 112 out of 168 = 67 per cent without), $\chi^2 (1) = 10.20$, $p < 0.01$. Children whose parents

Table 9.1 Proportional hazard analysis of factors associated with reunification during first four months in care

	Parameter estimate	Wald	Risk-ratio
Total sample			
Aboriginality	−1.62	5.05	0.20
Neglect	−1.01	6.21	0.36
Parental incapicity	0.77	7.68	2.16
Children coming into care			
Aboriginality	−2.21	4.76	0.11
Neglect	−0.89	4.57	0.41

Note
No significant predictors were identified for the children already in care.

had some form of incapacity also tended to be younger ($M = 9.25$, $SD = 3.04$ versus $M = 10.93$, $SD = 3.43$), $t(233) = 2.29$, $p < 0.05$. However, as implied by the univariate analyses, neither behaviour nor age was associated with reunification directly.

The significant predictors were entered (using backward elimination) into a proportional hazards analysis using the log-linear likelihood ratio as the test statistic. The final model retained neglect, parental incapacity and Aboriginality as significant predictors (see Table 9.1). As indicated by the risk-ratios in Table 9.1, Aboriginality and neglect significantly reduced the probability of reunification, whereas parental incapacity increased it.

Sub-group analyses

A similar series of analyses was conducted only for children coming into care for the first time. The univariate analysis showed that reunification was significantly less likely for rural children (3 out of 23 = 13 per cent rural versus 40 out of 106 = 38 per cent metropolitan), $\chi^2(1) = 5.19$, $p < 0.05$; for Aboriginal children (1 out of 21 = 5 per cent Aboriginal versus 42 out of 108 = 39 per cent non-Aboriginal), $\chi^2(1) = 8.04$, $p < 0.01$; and for those who were victims of neglect (7 out of 39 = 17 per cent neglect versus 36 out of 90 = 40 per cent others), $\chi^2(1) = 5.95$, $p < 0.05$. Follow-up analyses largely replicated the results obtained for the overall sample. Neglected children were again found to be significantly younger than non-neglected children ($M = 9.13$, $SD = 3.14$ versus $M = 10.74$, $SD = 3.40$), $t(232) = 2.54$, $p < 0.05$, and were also less likely to have behavioural problems (16 out of 70 = 23 per cent with problems versus 36 out of 90 = 40 per cent without), $\chi^2(1) = 5.94$, $p < 0.05$. In addition, Aboriginal children were found to be younger ($M = 8.81$, $SD = 3.49$ versus $M = 10.54$, $SD = 3.31$), $t(232) = 2.17$, $p < 0.05$, and were less likely to have behavioural problems (6 out of 21 = 29 per cent with problems versus 64 out of 108 = 59 per cent without), χ^2 (1) = 6.67, $p < 0.05$. It is important to recognize that this relationship between behavioural problems and reunification is confounded by age. Children who are in care because of neglect are more likely to be younger, and this age group also tends to have fewer behavioural problems. For these younger children, then, it is neglect rather than behaviour that poses the greater obstacle to reunification. No significant predictors were obtained for the children already in care at the time of the reference placement.

Probability estimates based on identified predictors

As previously indicated, the strength of hazard analyses is that estimates can be obtained of the probability of reunification at any point in time, and for any combination of scores on the identified predictor variables. That is $h(t) = q(t)e^{Bx}$, where $h(t)$ = the hazard rate at a given point in time, $q(t)$ is an unspecified period of time, and e^{Bx} = e raised to the sum of the scores for the nth variable (x) multiplied by the nth regression parameter (i.e., B_0 through to B_n, where n = the number of significant predictors). Using the model generated for the overall sample, estimates for reunification were calculated for every combination of scores on parental incapacity (0, 1), neglect (0, 1), and Aboriginality (0, 1). A summary of the resultant probability of reunification after four months (120 days) is described in Table 9.2. This shows that reunification was most likely for non-Aboriginal children who were not neglected and whose parents had some form of incapacity (probability = 58 per cent after four months), whereas the reverse combination of variables was associated with only a 2 per cent probability of reunification. The respective hazard functions associated with these two combinations are provided in Figures 9.1 and 9.2. Placing the number of days on the x axis, these graphs allow us to estimate the probability of reunification based on the two variables from 0 to 120 days after placement.

Table 9.2 Probability of reunification after 120 days, by parental incapacity, on the basis of different combinations of scores on predictor variables (total sample)

	No	Yes
Neglected		
Aboriginal	0.02	0.42
Non-Aboriginal	0.09	0.21
Not neglected		
Aboriginal	0.05	0.12
Non-Aboriginal	0.27	0.58

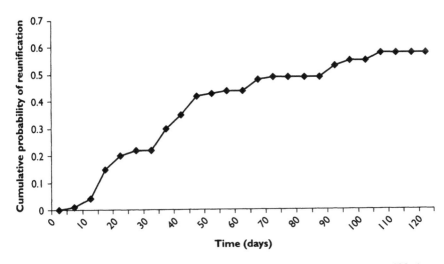

Figure 9.1 Factors associated with the highest probability of reunification in 120 days: non-Aboriginal, non-neglected and parental incapacity

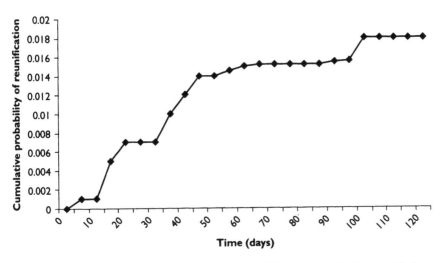

Figure 9.2 Factors associated with the lowest probability of reunification in 120 days: Aboriginal, neglected and no parental incapacity

An interesting finding presented in Table 9.2 is that children (particularly Aboriginal children) who were neglected because of parental incapacity had an increased chance of being reunified but that this probability dropped substantially when neglect was not associated with parental incapacity ($p = 0.02$ and 0.09). What this demonstrates is that neglect which is attributable to

Table 9.3 Summary of individual cases and reasons for their reunification

Reason for reunification	Gender, age	Physical or sexual abuse	Emotional abuse	Neglect	Parental incapacity	Child behaviour
Children coming into care for the first time						
Order expired	F 11	•	•			
	F 14					•
	M 14					•
	F 11	•	•	•		•
	M 5			•	•	
	M 13					•
	M 13					•
Returned to other parent	M 14					•
	F 8		•	•		•
	F 13		•			
	F 13	•	•			
	F 13		•			
	M 14					•
	M 9					
	F 7			•	•	•
	M 8				•	•
	F 7				•	•
Mother's physical or mental well-being improved	F 12				•	
	F 13		•			
	M 10				•	•
	M 4	•	•			
	M 9		•		•	•
	F 13	•	•		•	•
	F 10				•	
	M 8		•		•	•
	F 8					
	M 6				•	
	M 8					
	M 9				•	•
	F 7				•	
	M 8				•	
	M 15				•	•
	M 5		•			
	M 6					
	M 8			•	•	
Child's behaviour improved	M 15					•
	F 14					•
Other	M 11	•	•		•	•
	M 12	•	•			
	F 13					•
Children already in care						
Mother's physical or mental health improved	F 5	•		•		
Returned to other parent	M 11					•
Other	M 6		•		•	
	F 14				•	•
	M 14				•	•

Summary of reasons, n, (%) (n = 39 case files with relevant data available)

Mother's health or well-being improved	15 (38)
Other parent used	9 (23)
Order expired	7 (18)
Child behaviour and attitude improved	2 (5)
Other	6 (15)

short-term incapacity is associated with greater likelihood of reunification but the reverse is true for chronic neglect. In addition, Aboriginal children who were not neglected but who were in care for reasons other than parental incapacity had only a 5 per cent chance of being reunified.

This analysis was repeated for children coming into care for the first time, for whom neglect and Aboriginality were found to be significant predictors of reunification. Reunification was least likely for neglected Aboriginal (0.03), and non-Aboriginal (0.25) children, but highest for children who were not neglected (0.60 for both Aboriginal and non-Aboriginal children). Thus, for children entering care for the first time, reunification was most strongly predicted by the absence of neglect, irrespective of Aboriginality.

Summary of individual cases

The characteristics of children who went home within four months and the reasons for their reunification are summarized in Table 9.3. The description of cases and the explanations are simplified and restricted to cases in which information concerning reunification was available. Table 9.3 shows the relationship between the principal problems responsible for placement and the changes that led to reunification. The most striking finding is that reunification was very strongly associated with changes in the well-being or health of mothers. More than 40 per cent of cases were reunified because mothers (with or without support) were better able to cope after the children had been in care. This factor emerged even in cases in which other problems were also evident (e.g., neglect and behavioural problems), suggesting that these other factors were either symptomatic of or peripheral to the underlying problem. At the same time, the results also show that another 40 per cent of cases were reunified without any clear evidence of change in the status of the original parent (almost always the mother). Social workers were able to place 23 per cent of children with fathers, and a further 18 per cent of cases were closed only because the placement order expired and was not renewed. In several of these cases in which the expiration of the order coincided with sexual and physical abuse, social workers had placed reminders on the computer networks for the case to be monitored because of ongoing concerns about the child's well-being.

Predictors of family reunification in the medium to longer term

A similar series of analyses was conducted to identify the factors that were associated with reunification beyond the four-month point. A total of 37 children went home between four months and two years after intake, and these cases were included in a replication of the analysis described above. The first stage of analysis examined the relationship between demographic

Table 9.4 Proportional hazard analysis of factors associated with reunification after four months in care (up to two years)

	Parameter estimate	Wald	Risk-ratio
Aboriginality	0.91	4.54	2.49
Placement number	−0.07	4.04	0.93

characteristics, problems identified at intake and whether or not the child was reunified. These analyses again revealed a significant association between Aboriginality and reunification, χ^2 (1) = 4.73, $p < 0.05$, but in the opposite direction to that obtained above. This time Aboriginal children were significantly more likely to be reunified after four months (12 out of 35 = 34.3 per cent) than non-Aboriginal children (25 out of 142 = 17.6 per cent) were. However, consistent with the four-month analysis, parental incapacity was significantly associated with a greater likelihood of reunification (15 out of 49 = 30.6 per cent versus 22 out of 128 = 17.2 per cent), χ^2 (1) = 3.86, $p < 0.05$. Further analyses compared the children's placement history; psychosocial adjustment scores at intake, four, eight and twelve months; and the frequency of all forms of parental contact within the first twelve months. Only one significant difference was observed. Children who were not reunified experienced a significantly greater number of placements prior to intake ($M = 7.44$, $SD = 7.44$) compared with those who were reunified ($M = 4.64$, $SD = 5.56$), t (172) = 2.11, $p < 0.05$.

These significant variables were entered into a proportional hazards model using the same specifications as above, but no predictor was significant in the final model, so it was not possible to show how these variables influenced the probability of reunification across time. Thus, an alternative model was developed using logistic regression. This revealed two significant predictors: Aboriginality and the number of previous placements (Table 9.4).

As indicated in Table 9.4, being Aboriginal was associated with a 2.5 times greater likelihood of going home after four months, whereas with each 1 unit increase the number of previous placements was associated with a 7 per cent reduced probability of being reunified in this period.

General discussion

The results of this study share a number of features with those obtained in other American, Australian and British studies (e.g., Benedict and White 1991; Fanshel and Shinn 1978; Fernandez 1999; Pardeck 1984). Approximately a quarter of our sample had been reunified within four months of placement. In line with other studies (see Fernandez 1999 for a review), children who were already in care at the time of the reference placement and who had an ongoing history of placement had a decreased probability of reunification. This result therefore confirms the common finding that the probability of reunification decreases once children have been in care for some time. Furthermore, these children tend to be older and to have a higher incidence of behavioural problems, both of which are also factors that increase placement instability and the amount of time spent in care (see also Chapter 10; Bullock, Little and Millham 1993; Fernandez 1999).

Our results also provide further corroboration of the notion that child and parent characteristics reliably predict reunification within the first four months, and that the process of reunification in the short term can be distinguished by several key variables. Most reunification in this period fell into the passive category because of the role of extraneous and maturation factors (particularly changes in the parent's well-being or circumstances). For most of the children concerned there was never an intention to keep the child in care for very long. Although appropriate decision-making and social work practice is clearly required to facilitate and co-ordinate the process of reunification, the process itself appears to be governed largely by factors beyond the control of the child welfare system. In this study, such factors centred on the resolution of parental crises, such as release from hospital or prison, improvements in psychological health, and decreases in less severe cases of substance abuse. Indeed, in many of these cases involving the resolution of crises or releases from institutions, the return home could be predicted almost to the day. In short, early reunification tends to be associated with admission to care for reasons of temporary parental incapacity.

As shown in Chapter 5, the majority of children who enter care in South Australia because of parental incapacity tend to be younger and less behaviourally disturbed. Parental incapacity, age and neglect are all correlated so it is possible to identify a distinct cluster of younger children who are in care because of parental difficulties. This cluster of children is clearly the most likely to go home during the first few months of being in care and appears to fit the description of the 'early returners' described in previous research by Bullock, Little and Millham (1993). None the less, the study also identified characteristics within this group that decrease the likelihood of reunification in the short term. These include being Aboriginal and being a victim of neglect. Given the history of maltreatment and the ongoing controversy surrounding the so-called 'stolen generation', the finding that Aboriginality is associated with a reduced probability of reunification in the short term is worrying, although not surprising. Previous Australian research by Fernandez (1999) found that Aboriginal children typically spend five times longer in care than non-Aboriginal children, and a number of overseas studies (e.g., Barth 1997; Wulczyn and Goerge 1992) have found similar results for minority children of African or Hispanic backgrounds. Thus, internationally, there appears to be a clear link between minority status and time in foster care. The finding that neglect was negatively associated with early reunification was also consistent with previous research (e.g., Benedict and White 1991). However, as is clear from the profile of cases described in Table 9.3, the role of neglect is largely context-bound. In some cases, neglect was a consequence of other problems such as substance abuse that rendered the parent incapable of providing adequate care. In such cases, there is a reasonable expectation by social workers that the alleviation of these problems and improvements in the ability to cope will decrease the risk of further neglect. It is when neglect is not readily explained by such factors that there are greater concerns. Finally, the results also indicate that short-term reunifications do not always revolve around the resolution of pre-existing problems. For example, some children went home only because it was not possible to extend legal orders. In some of these cases (namely, where there was no serious abuse), there was no urgent need to apply for a more binding legal order because the child did not appear to be at serious risk.

Chapter 10

The psychosocial consequences of placement instability

Introduction

Chapter 7 reported distressingly high levels of placement instability in foster care, particularly in the first four months of placement. The level of instability uncovered was surprising given that all jurisdictions these days strive hard to minimize it. In fact, concern over this issue can be traced back to the landmark study by Maas and Engler (1959), which alerted the child welfare field to the phenomenon of 'foster care drift'. In Maas and Engler's study and many others since (e.g. Barth and Berry 1987; Bryce and Ehlert 1971; Claburn, Magura and Resnick 1976; Katz 1990; Maluccio, Fein and Olmstead 1986), it was found that children who were placed in what was intended to be temporary foster care were often left there by child protection workers for years on end while the bonds between the children and their families of origin gradually atrophied. Of particular concern to Maas and Engler (1959) were children who literally drifted from placement to placement as one foster family after another tired of the behavioural and emotional demands placed on them by these children. In an effort to prevent foster care drift, the policy referred to in Chapter 1 of permanency planning insists that every effort should be made to return foster children to the care of their families of origin as soon as possible; alternatively, the children should be expeditiously adopted rather than left indefinitely in the unconscionable position of provisional family members.

This preference for expeditious adoption is therefore the result of disillusionment with foster care on two counts. The first is that family reunification is proving to be an unrealistic option for many children in temporary foster care, so these children would be better off finding a permanent home with adoptive parents; or so the argument runs. The second problem, which follows from the first, is that many children now 'drift' in foster care in the sense that they remain as temporary family members sometimes for years on end because reunification is unviable and adoption is very difficult under Australian law. The intuitively plausible assumption behind permanency planning is that impermanence is inherently harmful and therefore that foster children can reach their potential only if they are allowed to settle into a stable home as quickly as possible. Given the strength of this conviction, there is a surprising paucity of research evidence to support it. Among the few studies that have systematically examined the issue is a twenty-year-old study by Lahti (1982) which included children from a demonstration project and children from a 'regular' foster care service. After collapsing across programme type, Lahti found that the best predictor of child well-being was a cluster of variables related to the parent's perception of placement permanence. Irrespective of where the child was placed – with biological parents, adoptive parents or foster carers – the degree to which the child was seen by the carer to be entrenched in the family accounted for more of the variance in child well-being than any other factor. On the face of it, these findings lend support to the emphasis on placement stability, and this is certainly how Lahti interpreted her results. In her discussion, Lahti stressed the need for follow-up services 'to assure the stability of placement' (p. 569). It is important to recognize, however, that Lahti's predictor variables related to attitudes and perceptions, not to placement stability *per se*. Interestingly, this same study also found no association between number of previous placements and child well-being, or between length of time in temporary foster care and well-being. Taken together, then, Lahti's results may actually imply that the attitudes and perceptions of care givers are more important than the stability of the placement itself.

This chapter aims to bring much-needed evidence to bear on the issue of placement stability. We begin by examining the psychological outcomes of placement instability before going on to identify which children are most likely to experience it. As we shall see, the relationship between placement stability and psychological progress is not straightforward and depends to a large extent on the length of time over which it occurs. For this reason, we have divided our analyses into two main sections: (1) the experience of placement instability over a period of less than one year, and (2) instability for more than one year.

Placement instability for less than one year

At the eight-month point, three main placement groups could be identified: (1) those who stayed in one stable foster placement throughout the period (stable) ($n = 49$); (2) those who changed placement within both follow-up periods (unstable) ($n = 31$); and (3) those who changed placements between intake and four months but achieved a stable foster placement during the four- to eight-month period (unstable–stable) ($n = 40$). Ten children who were stable in the four-month period but subsequently became unstable were dropped from further analysis because of the limited sample size. A further 105 children were not included because they had either gone home or were in other placement arrangements at the eight-month point.

Table 10.1 Mean, (SD) scores for conduct, hyperactivity, emotionality for the overall sample

	Intake	4 months	8 months
Conduct (n = 104)	0.72 (0.50)	0.61 (0.53)	0.54 (0.48)
Hyperactivity (n = 101)	1.21 (0.65)	1.02 (0.71)	1.09 (0.68)
Emotionality (n = 105)	1.07 (0.47)	0.96 (0.51)	0.84 (0.54)
Social adjustment (n = 109)	3.01 (0.48)	2.98 (0.40)	3.04 (0.43)

Overall analyses

In the first stage of the analysis, mean conduct disorder, hyperactivity, emotionality and social adjustment scores at intake, four months and eight months (Table 10.1) were compared for the three groups combined using repeated measures ANOVA. This revealed a significant Time main effect for conduct disorder, $F(2, 206) = 6.47$, $p < 0.01$, for hyperactivity, $F(1, 200) = 5.50$, $p < 0.01$, and also for emotionality, $F(1, 108) = 9.75$, $p < 0.001$, but no significant change in social adjustment scores, $F(2, 216) = 1.13$, $p > 0.05$. As indicated in Table 10.1, when one considers the three measurements points together there is a general decline in conduct and emotionality problems across the two follow-up periods, whereas hyperactivity shows an initial decrease followed by a slight upward trend. Fisher LSD tests applied to the individual means showed that these overall trends did not necessarily translate into consistent improvements. Conduct scores at eight months were significantly lower than those at intake ($p < 0.01$), but intake and four-months scores were not significantly different. In contrast, hyperactivity scores were significantly lower at four months than at intake ($p < 0.01$), but there was no difference between four months and eight months, or between eight months and intake. Finally, scores on emotionality were significantly lower at eight months than at intake ($p < 0.01$), but no significant difference was observed for intake versus four months or four months versus eight months.

Group analyses

In the next stage of the analysis, 3 (Group) by 3 (Time) repeated measures ANOVA was applied to each of the three psychological adjustment measures. For conduct, there was a significant main effect of Time, $F(1, 104) = 6.77$, $p < 0.001$ and also of Group, $F(2, 101) = 5.70$, $p < 0.01$, but no significant Group by Time interaction, $F(2, 101) = 1.77$, $p > 0.05$. For hyperactivity, there was no significant main effect of Group or Group by Time interaction, $F(2, 98) = 1.90$, $p > 0.05$, although there was a significant main effect of Time (as described in the overall analysis above). For emotionality, there was a significant main effect of Time (see above), no significant Group main effect, $F (2, 102) = 1.94$, $p > 0.05$, but a significant Group by Time interaction, $F (2, 102) = 4.03$, $p < 0.05$. Finally, for social adjustment, there was no significant main effect of Time, $F (2, 212) < 1$, or of Group, $F (2, 106) = 1.19$, $p > 0.05$, or Group by Time interaction, $F (2, 212) = 2.00$, $p > 0.05$.

In the next stage of the analysis, simple main effects analysis was applied to each of the three dependent measures in turn.

Conduct disorder

Beginning with conduct disorder, simple effects analyses were undertaken both within time periods and within groups across time periods to identify the source of the interaction described above. The interaction has been graphically presented in Figure 10.1, which presents mean conduct disorder scores. Within-group analyses revealed no significant time differences for the stable group, $F (2, 76) = 2.10$, $p > 0.05$, but significant differences for the unstable, $F (2, 56) = 3.33$, $p < 0.05$, and unstable–stable group, $F (2, 70) = 4.69$, $p < 0.01$. LSD comparisons revealed that intake conduct disorder scores were significantly higher than four-month and eight-month scores in the unstable–stable group. In the unstable group, scores were significantly lower at eight months than at intake. Within-time analyses also revealed significant group differences at each point in time: intake, $F (2, 109) = 5.73$, $p < 0.01$, four months, $F (2, 112) = 7.05$, $p < 0.01$, eight

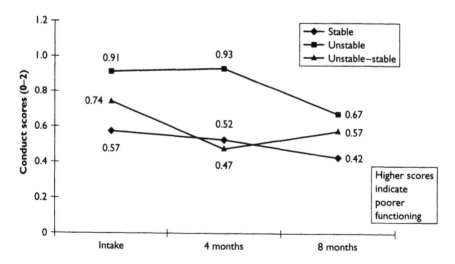

Figure 10.1 Mean item conduct scores across the first three assessment points

Table 10.2 Conduct scores, (SDs) restricted to children whose placements broke down because of their behaviour

Group	Age	Intake	4 months	8 months
Unstable (n = 17)	12.18	1.08 (0.52)	1.01 (0.63)	0.72 (0.50)
Unstable–stable (n = 14)	12.43	0.87 (0.38)	0.68 (0.45)	0.62 (0.54)

months, $F (2, 113) = 4.63$, $p < 0.05$. Fisher LSD comparisons showed that the unstable group had consistently more conduct problems at all three points in time than the stable group, and the unstable–stable group at intake and four months, but not at eight months.

The higher initial levels of conduct problems in the unstable group than in the unstable–stable group are also borne out by the reasons for placement change within the two groups. Seventeen (57 per cent) of the 30 children in the unstable group experienced placement breakdown as a result of their behaviour during the period compared with only 14 (35 per cent) of the 40 children in the unstable–stable group. Thus, in order to determine whether the trend identified in Figure 10.1 was a result of the different concentration of conduct-disordered children in the two groups, the analysis of conduct scores was restricted to children who experienced placement breakdown as a result of behaviour between intake and four months. Results of this analysis are presented in Table 10.2.

The data in Table 10.2 were analysed using a 2 (Group) by 3 (Time) repeated measures analysis of variance which produced a significant main effect of Time, $F (2, 52) = 3.51$, $p < 0.05$, but no significant Group effect, $F (1, 26) = 2.08$, $p > 0.05$, or Group by Time interaction, $F (2, 52) < 1$. Analysis of simple main effects was conducted within groups to determine the source of the overall main effect. This showed that there was no significant Time difference for the unstable–stable group, $F (1, 20) = 1.06$, $p > 0.05$, but there was a significant Time difference for the unstable group, $F (2, 32) = 3.51$, $p < 0.05$. Fisher tests applied to this result showed that the unstable group's conduct score was significantly lower at eight months than it had been at intake or four months. In other words, the unstable group's conduct improved during a period of placement instability, while the unstable–stable group showed no improvement over the study period. Importantly, both groups were also matched in terms of conduct scores at intake, $t (28) < 1$.

Hyperactivity

Within-group analysis of hyperactivity scores revealed significant Time differences only for the stable, $F (2, 72) = 6.81$, $p < 0.01$, and unstable–stable

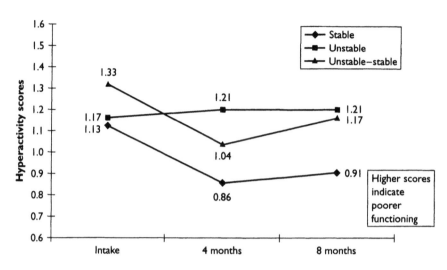

Figure 10.2 Mean item hyperactivity scores across the first three assessment points

groups, $F(2, 68) = 3.97$, $p < 0.05$. Consistent with Figure 10.2, analysis of simple main effects showed that the four-month and eight-month scores were generally lower than the intake scores for the consistently stable group, but that only the four-month scores were lower than the intake scores in the unstable–stable group. Within-time analyses revealed significant Group differences at four and eight months: four months, $F(2, 110) = 3.97$, $p < 0.05$, eight months, $F(2, 113) = 5.43$, $p < 0.01$. Fisher LSD comparisons showed that the stable group had lower hyperactivity scores at four months than the unstable group, and lower scores than both groups at eight months.

Emotionality

Within-group analyses revealed significant Time differences in emotionality scores for all three groups: stable, $F(2, 78) = 6.85$, $p < 0.01$, unstable, $F(2, 56) = 8.16$, $p < 0.01$, and unstable–stable, $F(2, 70) = 4.11$, $p < 0.05$. The consistently stable and consistently unstable groups had higher scores at intake and four months compared with eight months, whereas for the unstable–stable group intake scores were higher than four months scores only (Figure 10.3). Within-time analyses revealed significant Group differences at eight months only, $F(2, 111) = 5.46$, $p < 0.01$. Fisher LSD comparisons showed that the unstable and stable groups had lower emotionality scores at eight months than the unstable–stable group.

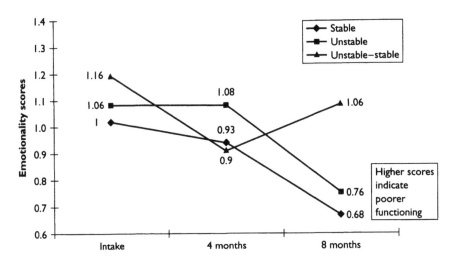

Figure 10.3 Mean item emotionality scores across the first three assessment points

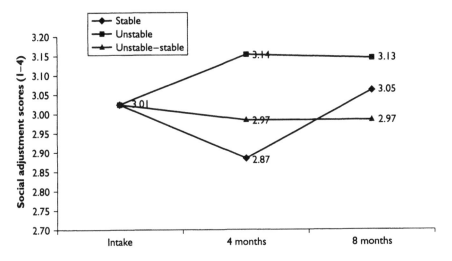

Figure 10.4 Mean social adjustment scores across the first three assessment points

Social adjustment

Within-group analyses revealed significant Time differences in social adjustment scores for the stable group only, $F(2, 89) = 4.17, p < 0.05$ (Figure 10.4).
A Fisher LSD test showed that the stable group's social adjustment score
was significantly lower at four months than at intake or at eight months.
Within-time analyses revealed significant Group differences at intake only,

$F(2, 111) = 4.11, p < 0.05$. Fisher LSD comparisons showed that the unstable group had higher social adjustment scores than the stable group at intake. At eight months, this advantage had disappeared.

Potential demand characteristics

The changes in psychosocial adjustment depicted in Figures 10.1–10.4 were also analysed in relation to change in social worker across time. This analysis was performed in order to test for the possibility that some or all of the improvements in child well-being noted above could be attributed to demand characteristics resulting from the same social worker providing repeated assessments. In the analysis, four groups were considered: (1) The same social worker worked with the child throughout and was therefore interviewed each time (SSS) ($n = 47$). (2) The same social worker was interviewed on the first two occasions, and a different social worker at eight months (SSD) ($n = 23$). (3) The same social worker was interviewed at times 2 and 3 (DSS) ($n = 22$). (4) A different social worker was interviewed each time (DDD) ($n = 24$). The results of this analysis are presented in Table 10.3.

Table 10.3 Mean, (SD) scores for psychological adjustment measures in relation to social worker changes

	Intake	4 months	8 months	Post-hoc
Conduct				
SSS	0.77 (0.48)	0.53 (0.50)	0.49 (0.41)	1 > 2, 3
SSD	0.71 (0.53)	0.67 (0.61)	0.60 (0.56)	ns
DSS	0.63 (0.46)	0.50 (0.44)	0.52 (0.47)	ns
DDD	0.70 (0.58)	0.76 (0.61)	0.58 (0.54)	1, 2 > 3
Hyperactivity				
SSS	1.17 (0.63)	0.88 (0.70)	0.87 (0.67)	1 > 2, 3
SSD	1.37 (0.51)	1.14 (0.77)	1.37 (0.61)	1 > 2
DSS	1.11 (0.75)	0.94 (0.69)	0.89 (0.68)	ns
DDD	1.15 (0.72)	1.07 (0.79)	1.20 (0.76)	ns
Emotionality				
SSS	1.14 (0.46)	0.84 (0.49)	0.86 (0.42)	1 > 2, 3
SSD	1.17 (0.37)	1.19 (0.52)	0.85 (0.62)	1, 2 > 3
DSS	0.91 (0.50)	0.70 (0.51)	0.70 (0.49)	ns
DDD	0.99 (0.54)	1.12 (0.42)	0.91 (0.66)	2 > 3
Social adjustment				
SSS	3.06 (0.49)	3.01 (0.41)	3.08 (0.45)	ns
SSD	2.93 (0.35)	2.99 (0.37)	2.97 (0.42)	ns
DSS	3.06 (0.30)	2.97 (0.48)	3.09 (0.35)	ns
DDD	2.94 (0.69)	2.93 (0.34)	3.02 (0.44)	ns

Table 10.3 shows that there is little evidence of consistent demand effects. Although conduct scores significantly decreased across the SSS group, no significant decreases were obtained (using Fisher LSD tests) for SSD (four months versus eight months), or DSS (four months versus eight months). Moreover, a decrease was also observed for DDD where the social worker was different on each occasion. For hyperactivity, there were significant decreases between intake and four months ($p < 0.05$) for SSS and SSD (consistent with the demand hypothesis), but similar changes were not observed for DSS (four months versus eight months). For emotionality, there was a decrease for SSS between intake and four months only ($p < 0.05$), but no other change was consistent with the demand hypothesis. As with conduct disorder, decreases also occurred in DDD (four months versus eight months, $p < 0.05$) where different social workers performed the three assessments.

In summary, then, results up to the eight-month point present a fairly consistent picture of the association between placement stability and psychological well-being. Although stable placements displayed a generally steady trend towards improvement, the other two groups did not behave as expected. Except in the case of hyperactivity, unstable placements also displayed gradual improvement across the period, whereas unstable–stable children displayed improvement while their placements were unstable, but not once their placements settled down. Importantly, these results cannot be explained by selection effects. This was clearest in the cases of hyperactivity and emotionality, where intake equivalence applied across all three groups. But, even in the case of conduct disorder, the pattern of results cannot be explained by selection. This conclusion follows from the analysis of conduct disorder scores that was restricted to children whose placements had been terminated between intake and four months because of disruptive behaviour. Although these children were matched at intake, only those children whose placements remained unstable throughout showed improvement between four months and eight months. Children whose placements stabilized showed no such improvement. It is also important to reiterate that the improvements cannot be explained by demand characteristics resulting from repeated administration of the same instrument to the same social worker.

Placement instability for a year or more

Instability after one year in care

By the twelve-month follow-up point, three distinct placement groups could again be identified: (1) children who changed placement in at least two of the three follow-up periods and/or were still unstable at twelve months (very unstable) ($n = 54$); (2) children who stayed in one stable placement throughout the year (stable) ($n = 35$); and (3) children who changed placements in one period only and were stable by the twelve-month point (moderately unstable) ($n = 26$). These three groups did not differ in gender composition, χ^2 (2) < 1, but there were significantly more Aboriginal children in the stable group (29 per cent versus 11 per cent in the other groups), χ^2 (2) = 7.47, $p < 0.05$. Children in the stable group were also significantly younger ($M = 8.63$, $SD = 3.30$ years) compared with children in the two unstable groups (M one period only = 9.65, $SD = 3.21$), and (M two or more periods = 11.57, $SD = 2.78$), F (2, 125) = 10.58, $p < 0.001$. The groups did not differ in number of placements prior to intake, F (2, 123) = 2.27, $p > 0.05$, but differed in the mean number of places in the first twelve months after intake. The mean number of placement changes for the twelve months across the three groups as a whole was 3.09 ($SD = 4.44$), with 1.69 ($SD = 1.01$) in the moderately unstable group and $M = 5.75$ ($SD = 5.24$) for the very unstable group. Analysis of the reasons for being in care showed that children in the very unstable group were significantly more likely to be in care because of some underlying mental health problem (31 per cent versus 10 per cent in the other two groups, χ^2 (2) = 8.47, $p < 0.05$).

Table 10.4 presents means (and standard deviations) of psychosocial adjustment measures for the three placement groups across all four points in time. The table also presents results of pairwise comparisons and effect sizes for statistically significant effects. As it was not always possible to obtain all measures on every child at all four points in time, Table 10.4 also records the number of valid scores obtained for each group at all points in time.

Adjustment scores were analysed using 3 (Group) by 4 (Time) repeated measures analysis of variance (ANOVA). In the case of conduct disorder, this procedure identified significant main effects of Time, F (3, 96) = 2.77, $p < 0.05$, and Group, F (2, 96) = 5.32, $p < 0.01$, but no significant Group by Time interaction, F (6, 96) < 1. Further pairwise comparisons showed that mean conduct disorder scores across groups at intake were significantly higher than at the other three follow-up periods. Scores at four, eight and twelve months did not differ significantly. Pairwise comparisons conducted across groups showed that the stable group had significantly lower conduct disorder scores than the very unstable group at intake and also at the three follow-up points. On the other hand, only the most unstable group showed significant and sustained improvement in conduct scores over the period.

In the case of hyperactivity, there was no significant main effect of Time, F (3, 89) = 1.55, $p > 0.05$, or Group, F (2, 89) = 2.12, $p > 0.05$; nor was there a significant Group by Time interaction, F (6, 89) < 1. Pairwise comparisons conducted within groups revealed no significant and sustained changes in hyperactivity across time, or significant group differences. However, inspection of the means indicates that the absence of statistical significance needs to be considered in the context of the small sample sizes involved. As Table 10.4 shows, the stable group recorded consistently lower scores than the other two groups at all four measurement points, with consistently moderate effect size differences throughout.

Table 10.4 Adjustment scores, (SD) broken down by group and time

		Very unstable	Stable	Moderately unstable	Pairwise contrasts	Effect size (d)
Conduct disorder		n = 48	n = 24	n = 20		
Intake	1	0.87 (0.48)	0.53 (0.48)	0.71 (0.53)	1 > 2	0.71
4 months	2	0.80 (0.59)	0.43 (0.48)	0.44 (0.35)	1 > 2, 3	0.69, 0.77
8 months	3	0.69 (0.49)	0.42 (0.50)	0.57 (0.50)	1 > 2	0.55
12 months	4	0.69 (0.49)	0.46 (0.48)	0.63 (0.49)	ns	
Pairwise comparisons		1 > 3, 4	ns	2 < 1		
Effect size (d)		0.37, 0.37		0.61		
Hyperactivity		n = 47	n = 21	n = 18		
Intake	1	1.29 (0.60)	0.99 (0.66)	1.31 (0.68)	ns	
4 months	2	1.11 (0.77)	0.89 (0.67)	1.19 (0.73)	ns	
8 months	3	1.22 (0.69)	0.92 (0.71)	1.20 (0.65)	ns	
12 months	4	1.13 (0.67)	0.87 (0.68)	1.28 (0.67)	ns	
Pairwise comparisons		2 < 1	ns	ns		
Effect size (d)		0.24				
Emotionality		n = 49	n = 22	n = 20		
Intake	1	1.10 (0.47)	1.00 (0.54)	1.22 (0.44)	ns	
4 months	2	1.05 (0.48)	0.94 (0.56)	0.92 (0.48)	ns	
8 months	3	0.84 (0.56)	0.76 (0.54)	1.11 (0.50)	2 < 3	0.67
12 months	4	0.88 (0.53)	0.68 (0.60)	0.89 (0.43)	ns	
Pairwise comparisons		1 > 3, 4	1–2 > 4	1 > 2, 4		
Effect size (d)		0.50, 0.44	0.44, 0.56	0.65, 0.76		0.34
Social adjustment		n = 50	n = 25	n = 24		
Intake	1	3.06 (0.52)	2.98 (0.53)	2.73 (0.61)	1 > 3	0.58
4 months	2	3.08 (0.33)	2.81 (0.55)	2.92 (0.46)	2 > 1	
8 months	3	3.11 (0.39)	3.08 (0.43)	2.90 (0.49)	ns	
12 months	4	2.74 (0.63)	3.01 (0.52)	2.88 (0.50)	ns	
Pairwise comparisons		1, 2, 3 > 4	3 > 2	ns		
Effect size (d)		0.56, 0.71, 0.67				

Analysis of variance identified a significant main effect of Time on emotionality scores, $F(3, 264) = 6.73$, $p < 0.001$, but no significant Group effect, $F(2, 88) = 1.46$, $p > 0.05$, or Group by Time interaction, $F(6, 264) = 1.39$, $p > 0.05$. Comparisons conducted at each point in time revealed group differences at eight months only. Fisher LSD tests showed that the moderately unstable group had higher scores than the stable group. Further pairwise comparisons conducted within groups revealed that all three groups experienced improvements in emotionality over the twelve months. Most effect sizes for the CBC analyses were moderate to large.

Finally, analysis of social adjustment scores revealed a significant Group by Time interaction, $F(6, 288) = 3.12$, $p < 0.05$. Analysis of simple main effects involving the comparison of scores across time within each group separately showed that the unstable group experienced significant change, $F (3, 147) = 8.23$, $p < 0.01$. Fisher tests showed that, although the most unstable group had the highest social adjustment scores at intake, they experienced the greatest deterioration in social functioning and scored lower than the stable group at twelve months, although this difference was not detected because of the limited sample size and power of the analyses.

Instability after two years in care

The focus of this final analysis was to examine the progress of those children who were very unstable at twelve months and who remained in the care system after two years. In this analysis, two-year psychosocial adjustment scores were compared with those obtained at the twelve-month follow-up and also at intake. When interpreting these results we should recognize that this sample selection is based upon the children's status at two years (in care), so that the means provided below differ slightly from those described above in Table 10.4 (the one-year and intake assessment points). Conduct disorder, hyperactivity, emotionality and social adjustment at these equally spaced intervals are shown diagrammatically in Figures 10.5–10.8.

Analyses were conducted using a 3 (Time) by 3 (Group) analysis of variance (ANOVA) with repeated measures on Time. The analysis of conduct disorder scores revealed no significant main effect of Time, $F (2, 146) = 1.98$, $p > 0.05$, or Time by Group interaction, $F (4, 82) < 1$, suggesting no significant change in conduct scores in the interval twelve months to two years.

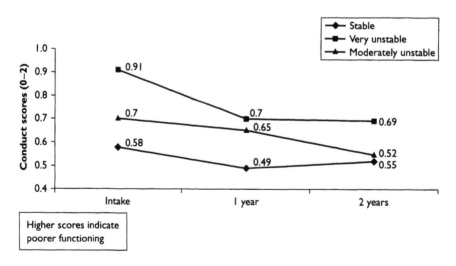

Figure 10.5 Mean item conduct disorder scores at intake, one year and two years

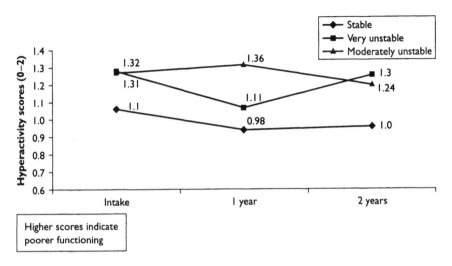

Figure 10.6 Mean item hyperactivity scores at intake, one year and two years

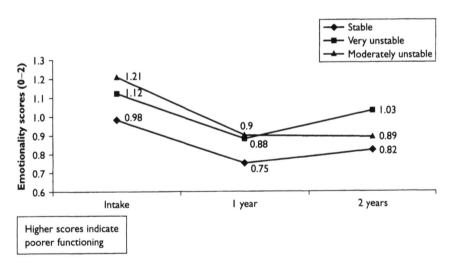

Figure 10.7 Mean item emotionality scores at intake, one year and two years

There was also no significant main effect of Group, although this was close to significance, $F (2, 73) = 2.89$, $p = 0.10$. Comparisons of scores across groups indicates that the unstable group scored significantly higher than the stable group at intake, but not at twelve months or at two years.

For hyperactivity, there were no main effects of Time, Group or interaction, and no significant group differences, largely because of the limited

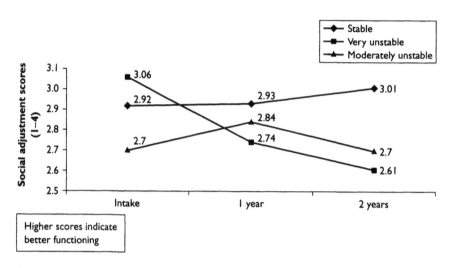

Figure 10.8 Mean item social adjustment scores at intake, one year and two years

sample sizes involved, but a trend towards poorer scores in the unstable group by twelve months. For emotionality, only the main effect of Time was significant, $F(2, 144) = 5.25$, $p < 0.01$. Fisher post-hoc tests revealed that scores at the twelve-month point were generally lower than at intake. Further post-hoc comparisons revealed that, at both twelve months and two years, scores for the two unstable groups did not differ significantly but that there was a clear trend towards improved scores in the stable group and towards poorer scores in the most unstable group at twelve months.

For social adjustment, there was no significant main effect of Time, $F(2, 204) = 1.28$, $p > 0.05$, but a main effect of Group, $F(2, 102) = 3.52$, $p < 0.05$. The Group by Time interaction was close to significance, $F(4, 204) = 2.17$, $p = 0.07$, and Fisher LSD comparisons confirmed that, although there were no significant changes in social adjustment scores in the three groups, the very unstable group scored significantly lower than the stable group at two years, after having the highest score at intake.

In summary, then, the results at two years show that there was a clear trend towards poorer psychological adjustment in the very unstable group as time went on. Whereas conduct disorder scores had stabilized in the very unstable group at twelve months, the moderately unstable group began to improve, so that, by the end of the study period, the very unstable group stood out as the most troublesome of the groups. In addition, the trend towards improvement in hyperactivity and emotionality that was evident within the very unstable group at twelve months reversed itself in the next period (twelve months to two years), while social adjustment continued to decline. Meanwhile, there was a trend towards improvement or at least stabilization of scores in the stable or moderately unstable group on all measures except for social adjustment within the moderately unstable condition.

A potential limitation of these analyses, of course, is that the groups included in the two-year analysis were actually defined at twelve months. As a result, the analyses do not necessarily tell us whether adjustment score variations genuinely covaried with different degrees of placement stability over the full two years. To elucidate this issue, a cross-tabulation of place-ment stability and group membership was conducted. This was achieved by examining the relationship between the two-year placement status of the remaining children (stable versus unstable) in relation to the three twelve-month groups. The association between the two variables was highly sig-nificant, χ^2 (2) = 30.11, $p < 0.001$, and the results showed that the pattern of placement outcomes for each group was maintained to the end of the second year. Specifically, of the 27 children still in care in the stable group, 24 or 89 per cent remained stable at two years; 18 of the 22 (82 per cent) of the moderately stable group were stable, whereas only 14 of the 46 (30 per cent) in the very unstable group were stable in care at two years. These results suggest some improvement in the placement stability of children in the moder-ately unstable group, but clearly show that the stable and very unstable groups remained very much intact across the two-year period. This there-fore confirms that the twelve-month to two-year analyses described earlier do provide a valid assessment of the psychological progress of the three placement groups.

Predictors of placement instability after two years in care

A final analysis examined the characteristics at intake that predicted whether children would be stable or unstable in care at two years. The first stage of the analysis involved a series of univariate analyses to identify individual factors that were significantly associated with placement stability at two years. Variables selected at this stage included the principal reasons why the child was in care (physical, sexual, emotional abuse and neglect), child disability, child mental health, parental incapacity, intake psychosocial adjustment scores, age and gender. These analyses uncovered only two significant predictors: gender and conduct disorder. Of the 49 girls still in care at two years, 33 or 67 per cent were stable in care compared with only 26 of the 60 (43 per cent) boys, χ^2 (1) = 6.26, $p < 0.05$. Children who were unstable in care also had significantly higher intake levels of conduct dis-order ($M = 0.98, SD = 0.41$) than those who were stable ($M = 0.63, SD = 0.63$), t (97) = 3.88, $p < 0.001$. These variables were then entered into logistic regression analysis with two-year placement status as the dependent. Both remained significant in the model. The odds-ratio for gender was 0.35 and

4.92 for conduct disorder. Using this information and the equation coefficients, it can be shown that boys with the maximum score on the conduct disorder scale at intake had a 91 per cent chance of being unstable if still in care at two years, whereas girls who scored only 0.1 on the scale (range 0.0 to 2.0) had only a 3 per cent chance of being unstable if still in care at two years.

General discussion

Taken together, these results provide only qualified support for the emphasis on placement stability that is evident in the permanency planning philosophy. Contrary to expectations, repeated placement disruption within the first eight months of referral into care was not associated with psychological deterioration. In fact, it was the group that started out in unstable placements but then settled down that displayed the worst outcomes by the eight-month follow-up. While it is conceivable that the apparent deterioration in this group may reflect temporary stresses in the transition to permanency, it is more difficult to explain the steady improvement of the group that was unstable throughout the entire eight-month period. After one year in care, our results began to present a rather more mixed picture. At this point, children in our sample could again be divided into three groups according to the stability of their placements at that time. When this was done, the predictable difference at intake in conduct disorder and hyperactivity between the stable and very unstable groups persisted throughout the twelve-month period. Moreover, the social adjustment of very unstable children underwent a moderate to large decline between eight and twelve months in care. Both of these results are broadly consistent with the permanency planning philosophy. On the other hand, only the very unstable group displayed significantly improved conduct between intake and twelve months despite being no different from the moderately unstable group at intake. Moreover, within-group comparisons demonstrated that emotional distress declined in all three groups over time. This latter result is particularly surprising, as it seems self-evident that protracted placement disruption should result in emotional distress. On the contrary, however, what our results actually suggest is that emotional gains are likely to be made by all groups up to the twelve-month point; it is merely that the greatest gains will be made by children in the moderately unstable group (see effect size comparisons in Table 10.4). Analyses conducted after two years in care show that, if placement instability continues throughout this time, it is quite clearly associated with adverse psychosocial outcomes. Not only did the trend towards improved conduct that had been evident in the very unstable group up to twelve months discontinue, but hyperactivity and emotionality began to deteriorate and social adjustment continued its decline. As a result, after a promising first year, children in the very unstable group ended the period significantly more hyperactive and emotionally distressed than stable children did, despite being no more distressed at intake.

In short, it seems that placement instability for a period of up to one year need not necessarily be associated with psychosocial harm; it is only when disruption extends beyond that time that problems arise. Naturally we do not infer from this that providing placement stability from the outset is not a worthy objective; only that it does not deserve to be the sole, or even the primary, objective of foster care policy. This would be to confuse means with ends and could lead to premature case closure. Ultimately, what matters most is the well-being of the child, and, regrettably, this objective may sometimes dictate that a child should be moved out of a placement for the sake of all concerned. When placement stability is elevated to an end in itself, there is an obvious disincentive to take this kind of corrective action. Foster children may need to change placement for all sorts of reasons and many of these reasons are positive, such as finding a foster home within their old school district or closer to their families of origin. Under these circumstances, improvements in psychological well-being are only to be expected. The weakness of permanency planning philosophy, then, is that it may impose placement stability prematurely via legislative or administrative fiat. Results in this chapter imply that foster care workers should be allowed the discretion to move children when there is both a need and an opportunity to do so. It is only when changing placement becomes a strategy for managing a child's unsuitability for conventional family-based foster care that damage is done.

In the next chapter we report on one group of children for whom repeated placement change was used in precisely this way. By the two-year point, these children were heavily concentrated in the very unstable group, yet they remained in the foster care system throughout the study period despite the fact that it had become apparent quite early on that conventional family-based foster care was unsuitable for them. These are children who were repeatedly rejected from placement because carers would not or could not tolerate their disruptive behaviour. As we shall see, when we restrict our analysis to this group of children, we soon discover a level of itinerancy and psychosocial distress that qualifies the majority of them as both homeless and traumatized.

Chapter 11

The serial eviction of disruptive children

Introduction

In this chapter we consider the progress of the most disruptive children in our sample. These children would probably once have been placed in institutional care but, because of the forces described in Chapter 3, find themselves these days in the foster care system. For the purposes of this chapter, disruptiveness has been defined as a minimum of two placement breakdowns due to behaviour over the life of the study. We set criterion at two breakdowns because of the high rate of false positives recorded in case files (see also Chapter 12). In other words, it was common for social workers to record 'disruptive behaviour' as the reason for terminating a placement when the situation was either more complex than that or was merely a case of incompatibility between child and foster carer. However, when disruptive behaviour was mentioned as the cause on more than one occasion, the problem of false positives disappeared and a sub-group of fifty children clearly satisfied the selection criterion.

A statistical profile of disruptive children

Overall, the disruptive group was older than the rest of the sample ($M = 12.26$ years, $SD = 2.33$ versus $M = 10.35$, $SD = 3.57$), $t(233) = 4.53$, $p < 0.001$, but membership of the disruptive group was not associated with gender, ethnicity, origin (rural versus metropolitan) or length of placement history. A second series of analyses examined whether the problems identified within the disruptive group at intake differed from the rest of the sample. This analysis showed that disruptive children were no more likely to be victims of abuse or to have physical, intellectual or psychiatric disabilities. As expected, however, disruptive children were more likely to be in care because of their problematic behaviour, $\chi^2(1) = 17.89$, $p < 0.001$ (86 per cent versus 53 per cent for the rest of the sample), and less likely to be in care for reasons of parental incapacity, $\chi^2(1) = 5.97$, $p < 0.05$ (18 per cent versus 36 per cent). Apart from age and problem(s) at intake, univariate analysis identified two other factors that distinguished the disruptive group from the rest of the sample at intake: conduct disorder and hyperactivity (see below).

All significant variables were then entered as predictors with group membership (0 = non-disruptive, 1 = disruptive) as the dependent measure in logistic regression. The log-linear likelihood was used as the test statistic, and backwards elimination was the method of variable entry. The initial model showed that only two variables remained significant: conduct disorder and age. A second model was therefore developed including only these variables. This model correctly classified 76.7 per cent of cases, and the odds-ratios showed that unit increases in age were associated with a 1.17 greater likelihood of being in the disruptive group, and unit increases in conduct disorder scores gave rise to a 3.88 times greater likelihood. The log-linear likelihood ratio was highly significant for both predictors ($p < 0.001$), and the final logistic equation was given by: 4.07 + 0.55 age + 1.36 conduct.

The probability of being in the disruptive group P(D) is given by $e^z/1 + e^z$, where $z = B_0 + B_1.X_1 + B_2.X_2 + \ldots + B_n.X_n$, z represents the linear relationship between the predictors and the dependent measure, B_0 to B_n, refers to the unstandardized regression coefficients, and X_1 to X_n represent the values of the constant (B_0) and significant predictor variables. Using this formula, it is possible to express exact probability estimates of being in the disruptive group based upon specific combinations of predictor variables. For example, if a child had a conduct disorder score of 2.0 (the maximum possible) at intake and was fifteen years old, that child would have a 73 per cent probability of experiencing two or more placement breakdowns as a result of behaviour. By contrast, a child of eight years with no conduct disorder at intake would have only a 5.6 per cent probability of being subsequently disruptive.

In summary, then, these results suggest that membership of the disruptive group is fairly predictable at intake on the basis of a combination of age and intake conduct disorder score. Interestingly, these same variables of age and conduct disorder also emerged in Chapter 6, where we reported on two discrete sub-groups within our sample. In that chapter, we found that the children could be described as either disaffected or protected. The disaffected group was older than the protected group and displayed more conduct problems at intake, while protected children were more often placed in foster care because of parental neglect or abuse. We therefore examined the relationship between these intake cluster classifications and the disruptive group which is the subject of this chapter. Chi-squared analysis showed that there was indeed an association between cluster classification and membership of the disruptive group. Of the 50 children who experienced two or more placement breakdowns due to behaviour, 37 (74 per cent) belonged to the disaffected group, compared with only 13 (26 per cent) who belonged to the protected group, χ^2 (1) = 8.20, $p < 0.01$. To calculate the differential likelihood of placement breakdown in the two groups, a logistic regression was conducted with placement disruption as the dependent measure (0 = not disruptive, 1 = disruptive) and cluster membership (1 = disaffected, 2 = protected) as the predictor. This analysis correctly classified 79 per cent of cases and found cluster membership to be a significant predictor of placement disruption (Wald = 7.83, $p < 0.01$). The odds-ratio was 0.37, indicating that children in cluster 1 (disaffected) were 2.70 times (i.e., 1/0.37) more likely to be in the disruptive group. Further analyses showed that this cluster difference applied to placement disruption more generally. Specifically, the disaffected children were three times more likely than protected children to experience a placement breakdown due to behaviour in the first four months in care (24 per cent in the disaffected group compared with 8 per cent in the protected group), $\chi^2 (1) = 8.20$, $p < 0.001$.

The placement movements of disruptive children

Table 11.1 summarizes the number of placement changes experienced by the disruptive group and the rest of the sample for each follow-up period in the study. A 2 (Group) by 4 (Time) ANOVA with repeated measures on Time revealed a significant Time by Group interaction, $F (3, 438) = 6.06$, $p < 0.001$, and also a significant main effect of Group, $F (1, 146) = 99.91$, $p < 0.001$. Fisher LSD tests applied to the main effect revealed that the disruptive group experienced significantly more placement changes during every follow-up period. Simple main effects analysis applied to the interaction showed that the non-disruptive group experienced a significant reduction in the number of placement movements ($p < 0.001$) based on the comparison of the four months and one to two year follow-up periods. (The one to two year period was divided by one-third to make it equivalent to the first follow-up interval of four months.)

The placement movements of the 50 disruptive children within each follow-up period have been summarized in Figures 11.1–11.5. Figure 11.1 shows

Table 11.1 Mean number, (SD) of placement movements experienced by disruptive and non-disruptive children

	Disruptive (n = 183)	Non-disruptive (n = 48)	Post-hoc comparisons
0–4 months	4.49 (4.29)	2.09 (1.69)	3.78***
4–8 months	2.58 (2.05)	1.48 (0.97)	3.59***
8–12 months	3.06 (2.51)	1.42 (1.09)	4.32***
1 year to 2 years	4.91 (4.24)	1.36 (1.13)	5.61***

*** $p < 0.001$.

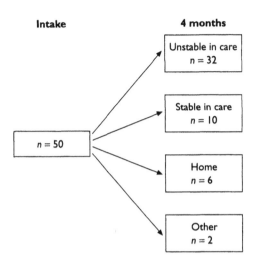

Intake   **4 months**

n = 50

Unstable in care
n = 32

Stable in care
n = 10

Home
n = 6

Other
n = 2

Figure 11.1 Disruptive children's placement movements from intake to four months

that most of the children in the disruptive sample experienced at least one placement breakdown within the first four months. Six of them were sent home, not because this was always the best option for them but normally because it was the only option. Moreover, Figure 11.2 shows that, by the eight-month point, only 5 of the 10 children who had been stable between intake and four months remained that way over the next four-month period. On the other hand, 13 of the 32 children who had been evicted from placement in the first four months settled into a single placement between four months and eight months. But, as Figure 11.3 indicates, most of these seemingly promising placements also broke down in the next period (eight months to one year), when 12 of the 18 children who had been stable in the previous period were evicted in this one. The profile of placement movements becomes even less stable during the longer period from twelve months to two years. As Figure 11.4 shows, only 3 of the 14 children who had been stable in care at one year remained that way at two years, and nearly all of the 24 children who had been unstable at one year were still unstable up to the two-year point.

The summary placement movements contained in Figures 11.1 to 11.4 are specified in Table 11.2, which shows the precise destination of each disruptive child over the period. It shows that, by the end of the study, only 9 (18 per cent) of the children could be considered to be living in a stable arrangement, as only these children had been living in the one place between the one- and the two-year follow-up. Moreover, 3 of these children were

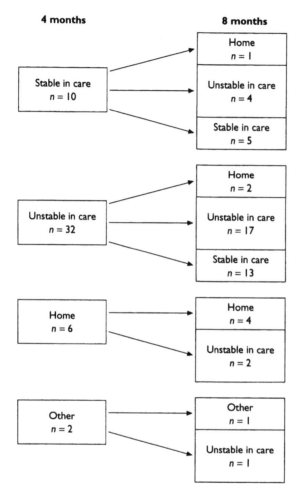

Figure 11.2 Placement movements of disruptive children between four and eight months

either in institutional care (*n* = 2) or living independently (*n* = 1). Of the rest, 4 were living at home and only 2 had found a stable foster home.

In short, the 50 most disruptive children in our sample, constituting 21 per cent of the total, endured two years of repeated eviction as one carer after another gave up and terminated the placement, or one alternative to foster care after another proved unviable. In the most extreme case (child no. 50), one child was forced to move home at least once every two weeks on average for the life of the study. This child and numerous others presented

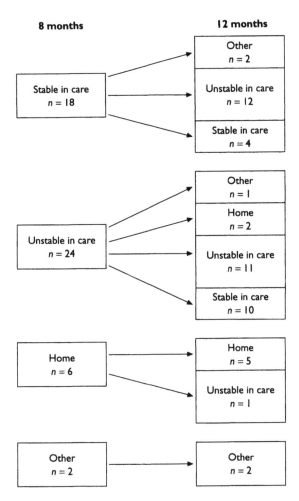

Figure 11.3 Placement movements of disruptive children between eight months and one year

in Table 11.2 could not truthfully be described as members of a foster family at all; rather they were homeless in care. This is a manifestly intolerable way of life for any person to endure, but particularly so for a child, whose need for parental affection and nurturance is a primal human instinct. We would therefore expect such children to display high levels of maladjustment relative to other foster children. This hypothesis is assessed in the next section which compares the psychosocial progress of disruptive children with that of the rest of the sample.

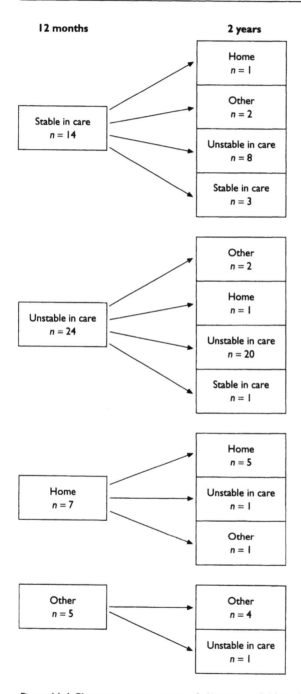

Figure 11.4 Placement movements of disruptive children between twelve months and two years

Table 11.2 Detailed placement profiles of each disruptive child

	0–4 months	4–8 months	8–12 months	1–2 years
1	F	FHFFR	RF	FFRFFFFRFFCC
2	FFFFH	H	H	H
3	FOM	OFMFMS	FCS	SCSCSC
4	FFFFH	H	H	H
5	F	FOF	FFFFH	FFFFFFF
6	FFFSYCYCSCO	OH	H	H
7	FIO	F	F	FI
8	FH	FFFFCC	C	C
9	FR	RFHR	RHFC	CF
10	F	F	FFF	FFFFCFFFC
11	F	F	FFFFF	FFFHFF
12	F	FFF	FFF	FFFO
13	FFFFC	CC	C	CC
14	F	F	FCFFHFFH	FYSISYSYSYSY
15	FFF	F	F	FCF
16	FHFFFFHFFF	FF	F	FFFFRFRFFC
17	FFFFFFFFF	FF	FFF	FFC
18	FFFSFCS	FFFFFFF	FFF	FCSCSCSCSCCSCSC
19	FFFFFF	FFFFFF	FF	FF
20	FF	FCCFF	FFFFFCSCSC	CM
21	FFFH	FHF	FHFFFH	H
22	F	FF	F	FFFFFFF
23	FF	F	FFFFF	FFHFFFFFHFFF
24	FOM	MFF	MFY	YFF
25	FCFH	FH	YYYYOY	YH
26	FF	FFF	F	FH
27	FFFFFFFCF	FF	FF	FRYC
28	FFHCFHC	CFH	FF	FH
29	FFFF	F	F	F
30	FO	F	FF	FHFHRO
31	FFF	FCFF	F	FF
32	FH	H	FFH	FFHOHM
33	F	F	F	FFFFFCSCSCSYSYSYSYS
34	F	FFFFFFFFM	MRM	FFOSM
35	F	FFFFF	FMFMFOFFFF	MCY
36	FFFRFFFRCMCR	R	RMFFFFMSFM	MYHYS
37	FFFFF	FFFFFFFHFY	YC	CYCM
38	FFFHF	F	F	F
39	FYFFFC	C	CF	FC
40	FFFFFFRFFFFF	F	FFFF	FF
41	FFMC	CC	C	C
42	F	F	FFF	FFF
43	F	FF	FF	FFF
44	F	F	FFF	FFFFFCF
45	FFFHF	FC	C	CFC
46	FF	FRF	FFOFFFFFF	FFFC
47	FFRFF	FYFFF	FFF	FFF
48	FOOF	FO	OI	I
49	FFFFFFFFFFFFFC	CY	Y	YSYSMSYSSSYSYM
50	FFFFFFFFFRFFFFFFFFFF	F	FFFFFFFFFF	FFFFFFFFFF

Key
C = Community residential; F = Foster care; H = Home; I = Independent living; M = Missing; O = Other; R = Relative care; S = Secure care; Y = Youth shelter

Table 11.3 Structure of psychosocial trend analysis

Period in care	Comparison(s)
4 months	Intake v. 4 months
8 months	Intake v. 4 months v. 8 months
12 months	Intake v. 12 months
2 years	Intake v. 12 months v. 2 years

The psychosocial adjustment of disruptive children

In the comparisons that follow, only those children who were in care at all relevant follow-up points have been included. Because disruptive children were, by definition, highly transient, they were often hard to find and were continually being assigned and re-assigned new social workers as the children moved from one region to another in search of a stable home. As a result, there was a considerable amount of missing data on psychosocial adjustment variables within our disruptive sample. Sometimes the child was missing when follow-up occurred, and sometimes the child's social worker did not yet know the child well enough to respond to our questions; sometimes the child had returned home; sometimes the child's new social worker had not yet been assigned to the case. In order to maximize the number of children included in our analysis, we needed to select follow-up points based both on interpretability and on available sample size. Judged according to these criteria, the set of comparisons presented in Table 11.3 yielded the best results.

After four months in care

A summary of the progressive adjustment scores of disruptive and non-disruptive children is provided in Table 11.4. A 2 (Group) by 2 (Time) repeated measures ANOVA was applied to each of these measures. For conduct disorder, there was a significant main effect of Time, $F(1, 141) = 5.73$, $p < 0.05$, and a significant main effect of Group, $F(1, 141) = 27.48, p < 0.001$, but no significant Time by Group interaction, $F(1, 141) < 1$. Fisher post-hoc tests indicated that the disruptive group had significantly higher conduct disorder scores at both points in time, and that scores for both groups combined had generally improved from intake to four months. Further comparisons showed, however, that this improvement was confined to the non-disruptive group. A similar analysis applied to hyperactivity scores revealed an almost identical pattern of results as for conduct disorder. Once again, there was a significant main effect of Time, $F(1, 137) = 4.69, p < 0.05$, a significant main effect of Group, $F(1, 151) = 6.13, p < 0.01$, but no

Table 11.4 Mean, (SD) psychosocial adjustment scores at intake and at four months

	Disruptive (n = 41)	Non-disruptive (n = 123)	Effect sizes
Conduct disorder			
Intake	1.00 (0.39)	0.61 (0.51)	0.87
At 4 months	0.91 (0.48)	0.47 (0.49)	0.91
Effect size	ns	0.28	
Hyperactivity			
Intake	1.31 (0.66)	1.09 (0.66)	0.33
At 4 months	1.25 (0.77)	0.90 (0.66)	0.49
Effect size	ns	0.29	
Emotionality			
Intake	1.15 (0.52)	1.02 (0.52)	ns
At 4 months	1.10 (0.57)	0.90 (0.48)	0.38
Effect size	ns	0.24	
Social adjustment			
Intake	3.15 (0.32)	2.95 (0.55)	0.46
At 4 months	3.09 (0.30)	2.92 (0.44)	0.47
Effect size	ns	ns	

significant Time by Group interaction, $F(1, 157) = 1.17$, $p > 0.05$. Post-hoc comparisons of the means in Table 11.4 indicated significantly more problematic scores in the disruptive group at both time periods. There was also a gradual improvement in hyperactivity scores over time, but this improvement was again confined only to the non-disruptive group ($d = 0.29$). For emotionality scores, there was no main effect of Time, $F(1, 146) = 2.38$, $p > 0.05$, no significant Time by Group interaction, $F(1, 161) < 1$, but a significant main effect of Group, $F(1, 161) = 4.08$, $p < 0.05$. Despite the absence of an interaction in the overall model, Fisher post-hoc tests revealed that the disruptive group was no more distressed at intake, but was significantly more distressed at four months than the non-disruptive group was ($p < 0.05$). A simple effects analysis, which compared scores across time for the two groups separately, again revealed a small ($d = 0.24$) but significant improvement in emotionality in the non-disruptive group, but no such improvement in the disruptive group. For social adjustment, the pattern of outcomes was different. This time, there was no main effect of Time, $F(1, 167) < 1$, no significant Time by Group interaction, $F(1, 167) < 1$, but a significant main effect of Group, $F(1, 167) = 7.01$, $p < 0.01$. Surprisingly, this effect resulted from superior social adjustment scores in the disruptive group at both times. Simple effects analyses revealed no significant change in social adjustment scores from intake to four months in either group.

In short, then, between intake and the four-month point, only the non-disruptive group displayed any improvement in psychological adjustment despite the fact that, on all three CBC measures, it was the disruptive children who actually had the greater scope for improvement. On the other hand, the disruptive children also displayed superior social adjustment (i.e., social relationships and social confidence) throughout the period.

After eight months in care

Table 11.5 summarizes the progressive adjustment scores of children still in care after eight months. These data were again analysed using repeated measures ANOVA, this time with three repeated measures for the Time factor. For conduct disorder, there was a significant main effect of Group, $F(2, 110) = 19.49, p < 0.01$, with pairwise comparisons again revealing significantly higher levels of conduct disorder in the disruptive group at all three measurement points. There was also a main effect of Time, $F(2, 220) = 6.44$, $p < 0.01$ but no Group by Time interaction, $F(2, 220) = 2.92, p > 0.05$. Simple effects analyses followed by Fisher post-hoc comparisons revealed

Table 11.5 Mean, (SD) psychosocial adjustment scores at intake, four months and eight months

	Disruptive (n = 38)	Non-disruptive (n = 92)	Effect sizes
Conduct disorder			
Intake	0.99 (0.40)	0.58 (0.49)	0.92
At 4 months	0.90 (0.48)	0.49 (0.50)	0.84
At 8 months	0.70 (0.53)	0.49 (0.45)	0.43
Effect size	0.62 (1 v. 3)	ns	
Hyperactivity			
Intake	1.35 (0.64)	1.13 (0.64)	0.34
At 4 months	1.23 (0.78)	0.92 (0.68)	0.42
At 8 months	1.30 (0.69)	1.02 (0.69)	0.41
Effect size	ns	0.32 (1 v. 2)	
Emotionality			
Intake	1.11 (0.50)	1.03 (0.48)	ns
At 4 months	1.06 (0.55)	0.91 (0.48)	0.29
At 8 months	0.92 (0.50)	0.83 (0.57)	ns
Effect size	0.38 (1 v. 3)	0.38 (1 v. 3)	
Social adjustment			
Intake	3.16 (0.31)	2.90 (0.57)	0.59
At 4 months	3.11 (0.29)	2.92 (0.45)	0.51
At 8 months	3.14 (0.36)	3.00 (0.46)	ns
Effect size	ns	ns	

no significant change in the conduct disorder scores for the non-disruptive group, but a significant improvement for the disruptive group from intake to eight months. Furthermore, the size of this effect was moderate to large ($d = 0.62$). The absence of any change in the non-disruptive group is no doubt due to the fact that this group could not have improved much after the four-month point without being remarkably free of conduct problems. For hyperactivity, there was a significant main effect of Group, $F(2, 106) = 5.07$, $p < 0.05$. Pairwise analyses showed that the disruptive group was significantly more hyperactive at all three assessment points. There was also a main effect of Time, $F(2, 212) = 3.06$, $p < 0.05$ but no significant Group by Time interaction, $F(2, 212) < 1$. Simple effects analyses followed by Fisher post-hoc tests revealed that the non-disruptive group experienced a significant reduction in hyperactivity from intake to four months which was not sustained to the eight-month point. For emotionality, there was no significant main effect of Group, $F(2, 111) = 1.79$, $p > 0.05$, nor was there a Time by Group interaction. In other words, the disruptive group was no more emotionally disturbed than the non-disruptive group across the period as a whole, but was more disturbed at the four-month point (Fisher test, $p < 0.05$). There was a significant main effect of Time, $F(2, 222) = 5.42$, $p < 0.05$, and Fisher post-hoc tests revealed that both groups experienced a moderate improvement in emotionality across the eight-month period ($d = 0.38$), although this effect was statistically significant only for the larger group (non-disruptive). Finally, for social adjustment, the only significant effect was a main effect of Group, $F(2, 117) = 7.31$, $p < 0.01$, with disruptive children again being more socially competent. Pairwise comparisons showed that this difference was, however, confined to the intake versus four-month comparison, and that by eight months the difference was no longer significant.

In summary, the conduct of the disruptive children at the eight-month point was no longer as challenging as it had been at intake, perhaps because of increases in the restrictiveness of placements as time went by or perhaps merely through maturation. Moreover, the previously inferior hyperactivity and emotionality scores of the disruptive sample also disappeared over this period. On the other hand, the superior social adjustment displayed by disruptive children at intake had also disappeared by this follow-up point.

After twelve months in care

A 2 (Group) by 2 (Time) repeated measures ANOVA was used to examine changes in psychosocial adjustment scores between intake and twelve months. Table 11.6 summarizes the mean (SD) for the four adjustment measures. There was a main effect of Group, $F(1, 110) = 24.09$, $p < 0.001$, which was due to the higher levels of conduct disorder within the disruptive group at intake and at twelve months. There was also a main effect of Time,

Table 11.6 Mean, (SD) psychosocial adjustment scores at intake and at twelve months

	Disruptive (n = 37)	Non-disruptive (n = 91)	Effect sizes
Conduct disorder			
Intake	1.01 (0.36)	0.58 (0.51)	0.99
At 12 months	0.79 (0.48)	0.49 (0.46)	0.64
Effect size	0.52	ns	
Hyperactivity			
Intake	1.42 (0.56)	1.08 (0.65)	0.56
At 12 months	1.37 (0.60)	0.99 (0.70)	0.58
Effect size	ns	ns	
Emotionality			
Intake	1.16 (0.47)	1.03 (0.48)	0.28
At 12 months	1.06 (0.53)	0.69 (0.48)	0.73
Effect size	ns	0.71	
Social adjustment			
Intake	3.09 (0.35)	2.89 (0.59)	0.43
At 12 months	2.56 (0.59)	2.96 (0.56)	0.70
Effect size	1.13	ns	

F (1, 110) = 8.31, $p < 0.01$, due to lower scores at twelve months than at intake. Although the Group by Time interaction was not significant, F (1, 110) = 1.81, $p > 0.05$, simple main effects analyses showed that the disruptive group experienced a significant decline in conduct disorder after intake into care, whereas the non-disruptive group had not. For hyperactivity, there was no significant main effect of Time, F (1, 106) = 1.40, $p > 0.05$, or Time by Group interaction, F (1, 106) < 1, but there was a significant main effect of Group, F (1, 106) = 12.39, $p < 0.001$, with the disruptive group scoring higher at intake and at twelve months. In the case of emotionality, there was a significant main effect of Time, F (1, 109) = 11.32, $p < 0.001$, with an overall improvement in emotionality over twelve months. Simple main effects analysis showed, however, that this result was confined to the non-disruptive group. As expected, the disruptive group scored significantly higher on this measure at both points in time, F (1, 109) = 10.89, $p < 0.001$. The pattern of results for social adjustment followed from the trend that was beginning to emerge at eight months. There was no significant main effect of Group, F (1, 115) = 1.11, $p > 0.05$, but there was a significant main effect of Time, F (1, 115) = 8.40, $p < 0.01$. As indicated by Table 11.6, however, this effect cannot be interpreted independently of the Time by Group interaction, F (1, 115) = 16.81, $p < 0.001$. The nature of this interaction was identified by simple effects analysis which revealed a significant decrease in social adjustment scores within the disruptive group. In fact, whereas the disruptive group had superior social adjustment at intake, the reverse was the case at twelve months, suggesting that deteriorations in social adjustment covary more strongly with placement disruption than the other adjustment measures.

After two years in care

The final series of analyses involved a 2 (Group) by 3 (Time) repeated measures ANOVA which examined changes in psychosocial adjustment at two years relative to the twelve-month and intake assessments. Summary statistics for this analysis are provided in Table 11.7. For conduct disorder, there was a significant main effect of Group, $F(1, 174) = 12.21, p < 0.001$, and Fisher tests confirmed that the disruptive group remained more conduct-disordered across the entire period ($p < 0.05$). There was also a main effect of Time, $F(2, 174) = 6.88, p < 0.05$, which reflected an improvement in conduct scores across the two-year period for both groups combined. However,

Table 11.7 Mean, (SD) psychosocial adjustment scores at intake, 12 months and 2 years

	Disruptive (n = 34)	Non-disruptive (n = 75)	Effect sizes
Conduct disorder			
Intake	1.04 (0.33)	0.67 (0.48)	0.91
At 12 months	0.82 (0.53)	0.55 (0.48)	0.53
At 2 years	0.72 (0.52)	0.54 (0.53)	0.34
Effect size	0.51 (1 v. 2) 0.74 (1 v. 3)	ns	
Hyperactivity			
Intake	1.41 (0.50)	1.19 (0.62)	0.39
At 12 months	1.38 (0.65)	1.03 (0.66)	0.53
At 2 years	1.33 (0.66)	1.07 (0.65)	0.40
Effect size	ns	ns	
Emotionality			
Intake	1.11 (0.38)	1.05 (0.48)	ns
At 12 months	1.08 (0.53)	0.77 (0.51)	0.60
At 2 years	1.07 (0.57)	0.82 (0.56)	0.44
Effect size	ns	0.57 (1 v. 2) 0.45 (1 v. 3)	
Social adjustment			
Intake	3.11 (0.36)	2.87 (0.68)	0.46
At 12 months	2.51 (0.61)	2.93 (0.55)	0.73
At 2 years	2.47 (0.46)	2.83 (0.53)	0.73
Effect size	1.18 (1 v. 2) 1.56 (1 v. 3)	ns	

although the Group by Time interaction was not significant, F (2, 174) = 1.13, $p > 0.05$, simple effects analyses revealed that the time effect was significant only in the disruptive group. In the case of hyperactivity, there was no significant main effect of Time, F (2, 84) < 1, or Group by Time interaction, F (2, 84) < 1, but a significant main effect of Group, F (1, 84) = 7.50, $p < 0.01$. Fisher post-hoc tests confirmed that the disruptive group was significantly more hyperactive at all three points. Importantly, there was no evidence of deterioration in this measure over time. Results for emotionality tell a different story. In this case, there was a main effect of Group, F (2, 86) = 6.39, $p < 0.01$ and Fisher post-hoc tests applied to this result indicated that the disruptive group was similar to the non-disruptive group at intake, but displayed significantly higher levels of distress both at twelve months and at two years ($p < 0.05$). There was no significant Time by Group interaction, F (2, 172) = 2.02, $p < 0.05$, but there was a significant main effect of Time, F (2, 172) = 3.20, $p < 0.05$, suggesting a gradual improvement in emotionality scores. But simple effects analyses confirmed that any improvement in emotionality was confined to the non-disruptive group ($p < 0.05$). The pattern of change observed for social adjustment scores was very similar to that observed at twelve months. Once again there was a significant Group by Time interaction, F (2, 182) = 10.29, $p < 0.001$, and Fisher post-hoc tests confirmed that the disruptive group had higher social adjustment scores at intake, but experienced significant and sustained deteriorations in social adjustment by twelve months which were maintained until the end of the two-year point.

Group comparisons after controlling for age

A potential weakness of the foregoing analysis is that comparisons between disruptive and non-disruptive children were confounded with age (see pp. 168–70). Thus, we may have merely reproduced the well-documented finding that teenagers tend to experience greater placement disruption than younger children, and tend to be less amenable to foster care. To address this issue, all analyses described above were reproduced selecting only children aged ten years or older. This allowed us to compare non-disruptive and disruptive children with almost exactly the same mean age ($M = 12.95$, $SD = 1.94$) for the non-disruptive group and ($M = 12.93$, $SD = 1.72$) for the non-disruptive group, t (148) < 1. A first series of analyses compared placement movements across the two groups and confirmed that the disruptive group experienced significantly more placement changes at every follow-up point. A second series of analyses compared psychosocial adjustment scores across groups and across time, and produced almost identical results to those described above. Thus, the differences in the outcomes between the two groups remained even when the two groups were matched for age.

General discussion

Overall, then, results presented this chapter show that the disruptive children in our sample were poorly served by foster care. Not only did they experience manifestly unacceptable levels of placement disruption, but their psychosocial development deteriorated over the period. In the first follow-up period (intake to four months), only non-disruptive children displayed any improvement in conduct disorder and hyperactivity despite also being better adjusted on these measures to begin with. Furthermore, disruptive children were significantly more distressed than non-disruptive children after four months in care. Surprisingly, social adjustment, which focuses on social relationships and confidence, was significantly higher in the disruptive group throughout the first period. By the eight-month point, the disruptive children who remained in care had begun to display quite sizeable improvements in conduct scores, and their relative disadvantage in hyperactivity and emotionality had also disappeared. On the face of it, these results seem encouraging and might even be taken to support persisting with foster care despite the short-term problems in psychological adjustment. However, by the eight-month point, the earlier advantage of disruptive children in social adjustment had disappeared, perhaps because their repeated placement changes had by then eroded the children's social networks and confidence. After twelve months in care, the adverse effects of repeated placement disruption began to stabilize. By this time it was clear that, although the behaviour of disruptive children had improved, they were also now significantly more emotionally distressed than non-disruptive children, and the social adjustment of the disruptive group had undergone a dramatic reversal since their entry to care. The psychosocial profile that emerged by the twelve-month point then persisted to the final follow-up point. In short, any improvement in the conduct of disruptive children during their time in foster care came at considerable cost to the children themselves. After twelve months in care they had fallen behind their non-disruptive peers in emotional adjustment and their social adjustment had atrophied to the point where they were now worse off than their peers, despite starting out with an advantage in this life domain.

Chapter 12

The views of disruptive children and their carers

Introduction

In the previous chapter, we looked at the predictors and the progress of children in our sample who experienced repeated placement breakdown as a result of their behaviour. We saw that placement failure was distressingly predictable on the basis of very few intake characteristics, and that children in this group were highly likely to bounce around foster placements until they were consigned to institutional care, ran away or 'aged out' of the alternative care system altogether. What these sterile indicators do not tell us, however, is what it felt like to be excluded and how the children explained the experience to themselves. Nor do the details we have presented so far tell us anything much about what, if anything, could have been done to salvage the placements. To answer such questions, it is necessary to talk to the parties involved, particularly the children and their foster carers. In this chapter we summarize the results of our discussions with disruptive children and their carers. We look first at 13 children in our sample whose placements broke down ostensibly because the child's behaviour was unacceptable to the carer. In these discussions, we sought to understand the child's reactions and, importantly, also to obtain the child's advice on what they and the foster care system can learn from their experience. We spoke next to foster carers of children who had been evicted from placement in order to benefit from their experiences as well. In all, we interviewed 19 carers whose case files had recorded that they evicted a child of the target age (ten to fifteen years) because of the child's disruptive behaviour.

The child's perspective

Information about the placement breakdown was collected via semi-structured interview schedule with 13 children aged between ten and fifteen years who had experienced at least one shortened placement ostensibly because the carer found the child's behaviour to be unacceptable. (Children under the age of ten years were excluded from interviews at the insistence of

FAYS.) One child had experienced two recent placement breakdowns and was interviewed about both. The total number of placement breakdowns examined was therefore fourteen. Interviews were conducted in the child's current home ($n = 10$) or residential institution ($n = 3$). There were 8 male and 5 female children, and their mean age was 12.75 years. Not all eligible children were available for interview, either because they were no longer under the care of the state or because their social workers considered that it would not be in the best interests of the child to relive the experience. All of the children interviewed had recently been excluded from a placement and had displayed multiple problem behaviours prior to placement breakdown. The behaviours in this sample included suicidal ideation, suicide attempts, animal torture, assault of a child resulting in medical treatment, numerous other physical assaults, repeated acts of property damage (for example, destruction of a set of dining chairs, holes punched in walls, garden furniture smashed), verbal abuse, running away, school refusal and threats of harm (including death threats) to the carer. In two of the cases, carer–child conflict over sexually suggestive behaviour by young adolescent girls led directly to the placement breakdown.

Interviews covered the following topics: (1) the circumstances leading up to the breakdown, (2) when placement problems first became apparent to the child, (3) the child's emotional response to the breakdown, (4) whether and with whom the child had discussed placement problems, (5) positive and negative aspects of the placement, and (6) whether any intervention might have enabled the placement to continue. The children were advised that they could have a support person present during the interview if they wished, but all elected to be interviewed alone. Interviews were conducted in a separate or private area of the child's current home or institution. The interview format was not followed in two cases, and not all questions were asked of all children. There were various reasons for these departures from the planned procedure. Four children were visibly distressed at some time during the interview and one interview was ended prematurely for this reason. Some other children appeared to become highly anxious at certain points in the interview and two young men were very reserved and difficult to engage. The format was therefore altered whenever necessary to minimize the child's unease.

Brief notes were taken at interview, more comprehensive notes made immediately after the interview, and a full record based on these notes was then written up. The printed interview records were subjected to content analysis, with each interview question being separately analysed. All responses were coded, a process which resulted in the creation of a number of nominal categories for each interview topic. The children's personal and placement details were obtained from the placement referral form, and in some cases additional information was provided by the social worker when approval to interview the child was sought. Carer details were obtained from the carer and/or from the relevant foster care agency, Anglicare.

Our interviews suggested that the children fell into two distinct groups: those who had disliked the placement and sought or welcomed the termination, and those who had liked the placement and regretted the placement breakdown. The former had few positive comments about their carers or their placements, whereas only one of the latter had anything negative to say about the placement. Cases will therefore be discussed according to whether the respondent regretted the placement breakdown ($n = 7$), or had disliked the placement and welcomed the breakdown ($n = 7$). (One respondent was in both groups. After the breakdown of a placement which he liked and which was the subject of his first interview, he experienced further instability in placements he did not like, and one of these placements was the subject of his second interview.)

Children who regret the placement breakdown

Four of the children who regretted the placement breakdown said that the carer had ended the placement because of their (the child's) behaviour. Unacceptable behaviours in this group included general non-compliance and sexualized behaviour; property damage and assault; repeated running away; and breaking curfews. One child told us that FAYS and the carer had made a joint decision to end the placement on the grounds of his behaviour (angry outbursts and property damage), and another young man said that, while the female carer wanted to keep him, her partner had insisted that the placement should end. According to another respondent, it was FAYS, not the carer, who had ended the placement. In this case, FAYS had stipulated that the placement would end if the carers did not enforce FAYS' prohibition on the child's association with certain adults whom FAYS deemed unsuitable because of drug-related activities. The carer had been of the view that it was impossible to stop the association altogether and she allowed limited, supervised meetings in her home. Two children told us that they had not been advised that their placement had been terminated until the day they were moved out. Three of the children said that they had not been aware of any problems in placement prior to termination. Two were unable to remember when problems began, but one recalled that problems began when she started to stay out late. One said that his placement problems started after the first week, and another after the first six weeks.

Three children said that, although they had liked the placement and wanted to stay, they accepted the fact that their behaviour (sexualized behaviour in public, repeated running away and property damage) made termination inevitable. One child told us that she had loved the placement and had not wanted to leave, another said he 'didn't like' leaving, one described himself as 'sad and unsettled', and another as 'pretty sad' at having to leave. One young woman said that she had been 'shocked' at being moved because she had not been warned that termination was even being considered and first found out she was leaving on the day she was moved. In fact, only one respondent had talked to his FAYS social worker about the placement change. This young man said that his placement had been terminated because of his repeated running away to search for his mother. His social worker had tried to arrange an access schedule with the mother but she was transient and drug-dependent and visits remained infrequent and sporadic. The running away therefore continued and the child accepted placement termination as an inevitable consequence.

When asked what they had liked and disliked about the placement, three children said that they had liked the carer, one had liked outings and shopping with the carer, one had liked cable television, and another said she had liked 'everything' about the placement. Only one child nominated a negative aspect of placement: the male carer. This young man reported that he had a very good relationship with the female carer but her husband was 'grumpy all the time' and never spoke to him. He said that the placement ended when the carers moved and the husband insisted that the child should not accompany them. This respondent also noted that the male carer had refused to speak to other children who went to the home on respite.

When the placement ended, two of the children who regretted the placement breakdown could not be placed in family-based care, and moved into residential care because there was nowhere else to go. One was told he could go to a family-based placement when one became available but he said that he preferred residential care, three experienced further placement instability in family-based care and one went to live with the friends who had been banned by FAYS.

Children who welcome the placement breakdown

Three young people in the group that welcomed the placement breakdown nominated their disruptive behaviour as the reason for placement termination. Two said that the placement had ended at their request, not the carer's. Another two said that they had told their social worker on more than one occasion that they disliked the placement and wanted to be moved, but that it was not until the carer requested termination that action was finally taken. Three children who had asked to be moved referred to the long wait before another placement was found. One said his social worker kept saying, 'next week, next week'; another said that it took 'about a month'; and the third commented that the wait 'seemed like years'. Two children could not recall when their placement problems had begun, but three identified problems at the start of placement, and one said that problems had become apparent six weeks into the placement. One child had foreseen problems as he had prior respite experience of the foster home, which he described as 'filthy'. He had been most distressed to learn (en route) that he was being taken back there, but when he protested he was told that it was the only placement available.

One child who had asked to be moved reported that he was 'miserable' when it eventually happened because, despite disliking the placement, he was sorry to lose contact with a friend who lived nearby. Of the other three who had asked to be moved, one said he would have run away earlier had the placement not been in an isolated area, one said he had been 'happy to move', and one said, 'My life began again'. The reactions to termination of the remaining three in this group were similarly positive.

Only one child had not discussed his placement problems with anyone, and some had sought help from several sources. Five approached their social worker; of these, three asked to be moved and the social worker's response had been to find a new placement. One respondent discussed her dislike of the placement with her social worker, who tried to negotiate with the carer. This respondent said that she had not gone as far as asking the social worker to move her because she did not want to give her social worker the worry of finding another placement. The young man who described the foster home as 'filthy' had telephoned his social worker but was told she was on leave. The duty social worker who took his call told him that nothing could be done as it was then the Christmas holiday period. The same duty worker also led this young man to believe that nothing could or would be done when normal business resumed. The child in question therefore took matters into his own hands and deliberately disrupted the placement by inflaming an argument with another child and assaulting him. (In similar vein, one child who disliked his placement commented that he no longer discusses placement problems with his social worker; if he dislikes a placement he simply behaves in a way that he knows will provoke the carer into demanding that he should be moved.) One respondent said that he prefers not to discuss his problems with anyone, and another had turned to a former carer who he hoped would take action to have him moved. Reasons given by the other children for not approaching their social worker included the belief that the social worker was not interested, and the conviction that there was nothing anyone could do to help. Two children had sought help from their parents (to no avail), two had spoken to a friend, one to a former carer and one to a respite carer. The two children who approached other carers secured termination of the unsuitable placement by, in effect, arranging their next placement themselves. In one case, the former carer took the child back and formal procedures subsequently legitimized the move. In the second case, while the social worker was investigating alternative arrangements, the respite carer agreed to the respondent's request to live with her permanently and opened negotiations with FAYS.

Two children in the group that welcomed the placement breakdown said that there was nothing good about the placement and a third responded that 'it was all crap there'. The other four children each nominated one positive aspect of the placement: going swimming; the family pets; being 'allowed to stay out all night' (in fact, the child used to run away to a former carer who allowed him to stay overnight); and a friend who lived nearby. Six children talked about being treated less well than other children in the home or feeling unwanted by the carer. For example, carers were said to have bought sweets, takeaway food or expensive clothes for their biological or other foster children but not for the respondent. An eleven-year-old girl spoke of being blamed whenever she and her foster sibling argued, and of her foster sibling leaving notes for her such as, 'Get out of here, you don't belong here'. She also said that the carer had confiscated her photograph album, both as a punishment and to discourage her from thinking about her family and consequently feeling sad (the respondent was in tears as she recounted these aspects of placement). A respondent who said she had always felt unwanted by the carer told us that the carer imposed an unreasonable weekday curfew, and that she had been given an excessive number of household chores and babysitting which left her with little free time (this respondent was also in tears as she recalled her time in that placement). The young man who had not wanted to go to the placement at all objected to the fact that the carers' cats lived inside and shed hair throughout the house, including on his bed. His objection had not been to the cats, which he liked, but to the state of the house, which he described as 'a dump'. The problem had been exacerbated by the fact that the carer forbade him to use the washing machine or vacuum cleaner. He said he tried to avoid eating prepared food by spending his pocket money on packet food. This young man was also visibly very distressed as he talked about his time in that placement. One respondent said that his carers did not care about him: when asked why he had reached that conclusion, he said that the carers did not give him pocket money.

Six of the children who disliked their placements stated clearly that no intervention would have enabled them to stay in the placement; they disliked the placement and wanted to leave. The seventh, the girl who had been unhappy because of inequitable treatment and confiscation of her photo album, said that she might have been able to stay if the carers had been 'nice' to her. Five children moved to stable placements and two went to new placements from which they ran away. Two of the children were vehemently negative about foster care, one describing it as 'worse than hell', and the other as 'a load of shit'. One said that 'foster care is no good for kids', and added that 'parents should make it so that kids can live with them'. There were two positive comments: one young man described living in his current placement as 'like being royalty', and another said, 'some places are good and some places are bad'. Other comments related to a preference for other children in the home; the difficulty of changing schools and leaving friends when a placement ends; the need for social workers to listen to and do something about children's problems; the need for children to meet prospective carers and to have a say in where they are placed; a one-month trial period for all new placements; and regular inspection of foster homes to ensure that standards of care and hygiene are met.

The carer's perspective

Information from carers in our study cohort who were said to have terminated placements because of the child's behaviour was also obtained via semi-structured interview. As previously indicated, the sample comprised 19 carers of children between the ages of ten and fifteen years who terminated placements and who agreed to be interviewed about the experience. An additional 3 carers were approached but declined to participate. All but one of the carers interviewed were female, although in 11 of the cases there was also a male partner in the household. Initial contact with respondents was by way of a letter which outlined the purpose of the study and advised that a researcher would telephone to discuss participation. Data were gathered via a semi-structured interview schedule which was designed to elicit information about: (1) the placement, (2) factors that contributed to the breakdown, (3) any specific incident that precipitated the breakdown, (4) the circumstances of the breakdown, (5) support available to the carer when problems began to emerge, and (6) the carer's response to the breakdown. The interview also assessed the potential for the placement to continue.

Brief notes were taken at interview, more comprehensive notes were made immediately after the interview and a full record based on these notes was then written up. As for the children, carers fell into one of two categories: placements that carers regarded as untenable ($n = 10$) and placements that were potentially salvageable ($n = 9$). A placement was regarded as untenable if the carer retained the view that the placement could not and would not be reconsidered. Placements were considered to be potentially salvageable if respondents stated that they had made the decision to end the placement precipitately and later regretted it, or if they stated that they would be prepared or would like to have the young person back in care, or if they identified an intervention which would have enabled the placement to continue. The responses of carers in potentially salvageable placements will be discussed first, followed by responses of carers from untenable placements.

Carers from potentially salvageable placements

Two respondents who regarded the placement as potentially salvageable actually denied that they had asked for the placement to be terminated. Both agreed that the child's behaviour had been disruptive but maintained that FAYS had ended the placement, in one case to avoid providing additional services, and in the other to facilitate reunification. These carers said that they and the child had been distressed when the placement ended. According to two other carers, their placements might have been maintained if FAYS had delegated more decision-making authority to them. Examples of social worker involvement which respondents perceived as unnecessary interference concerned the type of Life Story Book the child was permitted to keep, and whether or not the child could spend a weekend away on respite. There were two cases in which respondents had threatened the child that, if a certain behaviour recurred, placement would be terminated. When the behaviour was repeated, they believed they had no option but to carry out the threat; however, they subsequently regretted the outcome. Similarly, two respondents made the decision to end the placement during a highly emotional argument with the child. In these cases FAYS complied and removed the child, to the carers' subsequent regret. Two carers were unable to specify when problems began, but two had noticed problems immediately, and four had been aware of problems within the first three months of placement. One respondent who had cared for the child for many years said that problems began in the last twelve months of placement. Six carers had approached FAYS prior to placement breakdown and, of these, two had high praise for the support they received. The other four reported responses ranging from no help at all to more frequent visits by the social worker. Three respondents approached Anglicare for help and said that they had been well supported emotionally but that no practical assistance resulted. In most cases, the response to the termination request was swift removal of the child.

When asked how they felt at the placement ending, carers from salvageable placements gave the following answers: 'devastated', 'terrible', 'angry, upset and frustrated . . . in tears', 'it was the hardest thing I've ever done . . . terrible', 'pretty bad . . . in my heart I wanted him back', 'relieved and saddened', 'upset', 'sad but angry at the time', and 'angry'. The latter response was due to the respondent's belief that FAYS had been responsible for the breakdown by undermining her parental authority. Five respondents expressed their hope that the child would eventually return to their care.

When asked to nominate the positive aspects of the placement, all respondents in the salvageable group spoke of their positive relationship with the child, for example: 'we loved each other', 'I have a soft spot for that kid', 'a very loving kid . . . I could give him love but he needed attention and guidance', 'he's a lovable little boy', 'we loved having him', 'she was loving'. The two respondents who ended long-term placements (eight and ten years) said that they had considered the child to be part of their family and maintained that they had treated the child as they did their biological children.

Every carer nominated one or two interventions as having the potential to save the placement. Specifically, they called for more respite, immediate crisis response service, a child mentor, child counselling, and information and education about managing an adolescent. Two respondents who had ended long-term placements (eight and ten years) called for less interference from FAYS, alleging that the social worker had undermined their parenting and discipline practices by emphasizing to the young person that FAYS was the legal guardian and that foster carers had no authority to make decisions on the child's behalf, and by taking the child's part in disagreements that should have been resolved within the family. These two respondents subsequently left fostering altogether.

Carers from untenable placements

In 6 of the 10 untenable placements, the carers stated that the decision to end the placement had been made solely on the grounds of safety. These carers judged that a particular behaviour by the foster child posed an unacceptable risk to members of the household. The behaviours included physical assault, fire-setting and sexual activity with another foster child, and a male adolescent silently entering the bedrooms of females in the house while they were sleeping and watching them from the foot of the bed. One respondent had been repeatedly assaulted by the child but attributed the placement breakdown to the effects on her health of verbal abuse by the child. In the months preceding the breakdown, this carer had become increasingly concerned as the symptoms of her chronic medical condition grew more severe. She also reported that she felt anxious and depressed, dreaded going home and spent as much time as possible locked in her bedroom to avoid interacting with the child. When the child left, the respondent notified Anglicare that she would be unavailable for at least six months. This request to end placement was also categorized as being on the grounds of safety.

The three respondents who had ended a placement on grounds other than safety gave the following reasons: (1) frequent verbal aggression, (2) verbal abuse, and (3) refusal to comply with age-appropriate restrictions and discovering that the young person planned to steal the carer's car. In this latter case, safety was a secondary consideration as the respondent lives on a farm and the car is the family's only means of transport to the nearest town. In this untenable group, therefore, safety was the primary consideration in seven cases and a secondary consideration in one case.

Five respondents noticed problems immediately, and a further 3 were aware of problems within the first three months. One noticed problems towards the end of placement, another was uncertain about when problems began. Three respondents had asked FAYS for help, and two approached their Anglicare support worker for help with placement problems. They reported that these requests resulted at best in telephone support for the carer or an existing mentor talking to the child and, at worst, no help at all because there was no allocated social worker. Most requests for termination were answered by prompt removal of the child. When asked how they felt when the child was removed, responses from carers in untenable placements included: 'relieved but disappointed', 'sad . . . and relieved', 'happy', 'disappointed for [child] . . . she shot herself in the foot', 'good . . . nobody liked her at all', '[I] don't like to kick kids out', 'relieved', 'positive, a new start for [child]', 'relieved' and 'angry . . . glad to see her go'. Despite this, two of the respondents spoke positively of the child: 'He could be really nice . . .

pleasant', and 'friendly', and most spoke of the benefits they believed the child had derived from the placement. Typical responses were: other foster children in the placement had stopped the child from stealing; the child's academic performance and his relationship with his mother had improved; the child had enjoyed the placement; the child was clean and tidy and got on well with the other foster child in the home; the child's appetite and weight had increased. One carer from the untenable group who clearly disliked the child (at one stage she referred to her as 'that bitch') could find nothing positive to say about the child or the placement.

Five of the carers from untenable placements could think of nothing that might have saved the placement, one was unsure whether an agency crisis response might have caused her to reconsider her decision, and two identified interventions that might have saved the placement. One believed that, had her behaviour management plan been implemented, the violent incident which led to her ending the placement would have been averted. The same carer nominated better pre-placement preparation, by which she meant greater clarity concerning the terms under which she cared for and worked with the child. She had also been frustrated by disputes with FAYS over aspects of the day-to-day care of the child, for example being criticized over the type of meal she provided. She summarized the situation this way: 'FAYS has all the authority, kids have all the rights, and carers have all the responsibility.' This respondent left fostering altogether. The other carer who nominated better placement preparation stated that, had she known more about the child, she would have managed her differently. In fact, except for the two relative carers, all carers in both the salvageable and the untenable groups stated that they had received insufficient information and, for many, this was seen as a major problem about which they were eager to speak and provide examples. There were frequent references to the practice of 'stretching', that is, providing inadequate or incorrect information in order to secure a placement. Specifically, respondents referred to pre-placement questions being ignored, being told 'downright lies', being told only the 'bare essentials' and information being 'coloured' or withheld in an attempt to influence the respondent to agree to a proposed placement. For example, the carer of a boy who had displayed multiple extreme behaviours was told only that his relationship with his mother was poor and that the placement goal was reunification. Pre-placement information about a child who had unpredictable violent outbursts during which she assaulted carers and caused extensive property damage consisted of advice that the child had a history of placement breakdown and 'behavioural issues'. Carers expressed concern that ignorance of the child's background and circumstances compromised the care they could provide and their ability to be sensitive to a child's particular needs or problems.

The following six cases illustrate problems that arose as a result of inadequate or incomplete pre-placement information, or where the shortage of carers rather than the needs of the child dictated where a child was placed. Cases 1 and 2 are from the untenable group, and cases 3 to 5 are from the salvageable group. The sixth case involves a carer who ended placement on the grounds of her deteriorating health: it relates to a subsequent placement, not the placement which was the subject of the interview.

(1) One carer was reluctant to take a fourteen-year-old girl who she believed had been involved in theft. The respondent agreed to an emergency placement for a few nights but it was five weeks before another placement was eventually found, at the carer's insistence. During this placement the girl was living in a home where, in the respondent's words, 'everybody hated her'. It was also said that the girl cried when reprimanded.

(2) A carer ended a placement after the child disabled the smoke alarm and set a fire in the house. Pre-placement information made no mention of the child's history of fire-setting. One of the carer's close relatives had recently died in a house fire.

(3) In one relative carer arrangement, an adolescent shared a bedroom in a small house with four much younger children. Problems of lack of space and privacy were exacerbated by differences in bed-time, homework and leisure activity.

(4) A major factor in a carer's decision to end the placement of a thirteen-year-old girl was the respondent's discomfort with the girl's manner of dressing, which she described as 'provocative', and her possible sexual activity. The girl had a history of physical and sexual abuse, parental and extended family rejection, self-mutilation, running away and sexualized behaviour.

(5) A newly placed toddler screamed and appeared terrified when the carer attempted to bath her. The carer subsequently discovered that the child had been abused in the bath by a family member.

(6) A carer in the untenable group decided to withdraw from fostering for at least six months but was approached less than three months later and persuaded to accept a child for an emergency placement. She reluctantly agreed, despite the fact that the home to which she had recently moved had only one bedroom and there was no spare bed. The child slept in a sleeping bag in the living room.

Finally, carers were invited to make general comments on anything at all relevant to placement breakdown or foster care. In response, five referred to inadequate pre-placement information, and three noted that the system is hopelessly under-resourced, which results in children not receiving necessary services, for example mentors or counselling.

General discussion

Our discussions with disruptive children and their carers revealed numerous instances of poor social work practice, including inadequate preparation of carers, poor communication with children and carers, and inadequate consultation. Undoubtedly the overriding theme running through our interviews, however, was the depth of unhappiness felt by most children and their foster carers when placements break down. No matter how short a time the placement had lasted, almost all children and carers had entered into the relationship hoping that the child would become a happy and loved member of the family. When the relationship abruptly ended, most children felt rejected, even if they were relieved to be going; and most carers felt the grief or at least the failure that parents do when their children defy or spurn them. Significantly, the young people who were moved from a placement they liked fared considerably worse than those who were moved from a placement they disliked. Of those who disliked their placement, two ran away but five found a stable home. On the other hand, seven young people who were moved from foster placements in which they wanted to stay ended up in institutional care, or living in unstable or unsafe placements. These contrasting outcomes suggest that expeditious termination of a placement with which a child or carer is not happy may be the most sound intervention (see also Chapter 9) and, conversely, that early intervention to address problems developing in an otherwise promising placement should be a priority. Given the small and possibly unrepresentative sample, it is impossible to know the extent to which our findings apply to the population of disruptive children in foster care, but the fact that at least 13 children under state protection have collectively experienced such despair, is sufficient grounds for alarm. A number of the carers continued to mourn the loss of the child, and, even among those carers who were pleased to see the back of the child, there was regret that everyone involved had to be exposed to such upheaval.

In view of the distress caused by placement breakdown, then, it hardly needs stating that everything possible needs to be done to avoid evicting children from foster placements. And, as suggested at the outset of this book (see Chapter 1) and at various points since then, this is likely to mean not placing certain children in conventional foster care at all, whatever may be the supposed benefits of traditional family life. We will return this issue in the following chapter.

Chapter 13

Myths and legends in foster care

Introduction

Probably the most oft-repeated refrain in the review of the literature that appeared in Chapters 1 and 2 of this book was that there is currently insufficient empirical evidence on which to build outcome-based foster care services. Indeed, Part I of the book actually began life with the title 'Best Practice in Foster Care' but this had to be altered when it became clear to us that there is simply too little evidence to justify such a sanguine claim. A feature of the existing literature is that much of it is descriptive rather than evaluative; research studies typically involve small, unrepresentative samples and many are correlational in nature. Despite this, writers and practitioners consistently make assertions as if there were no ambiguity about the causal mechanisms underlying statistical associations. It is accepted practice wisdom, for example, that parental visiting produces better outcomes and that kinship care improves permanency, when all that has ever been demonstrated is that such variables are associated. Controlled outcome evaluations are therefore urgently needed before the facts of best-practice foster care can be separated from the fiction. In saying this, we recognize that the best that is likely to be possible is quasi-experimentation because there are very formidable practical and ethical obstacles to randomized controlled trials in the foster care field. In order to decide once and for all between the protagonists and the detractors of kinship care, for example (see Chapter 2), large numbers of children would need to be randomly assigned to kin and non-kin care so that the short- and long-term effects on 'subjects' could be dispassionately monitored. The number of children in such a study would also need to be large enough to deal with the many sources of 'error' that would inevitably confound interpretation of between-group differences in small samples. We trust, of course, that such an experiment would be judged by ethics committees everywhere to be unconscionable on grounds of human rights, long before its feasibility were ever seriously examined. But, even if the impediments to definitive outcome studies prove to be insuperable, the issue is not resolved by lowering the standard of evidence required for satisfactory explanation. The only alternatives to empirically derived practice standards are myths and legends; and myths and legends provide a very shaky foundation for complex human service systems. In the remainder of this chapter, we examine some of the more common myths in foster care that have been encountered in the course of this book and we explore the implications of our findings for each of them.

Myth 1: Foster care is in crisis

Foster care is in crisis; or so it has been claimed by a procession of contemporary scholars (e.g., Courtney 1995b; Curtis, Dale and Kendall 1999) and popular writers (e.g., Australian Broadcasting Corporation 1999; British Broadcasting Corporation News 1999, 2000; McLean 1999; Roche 2000; Teishroeb 1999). If you enter the term 'foster care crisis' into an internet search, you will turn up literally hundreds of reports, newspaper articles and opinion pieces on the subject. Often bearing nothing but the flimsiest of anecdotal evidence, writers and social commentators alike seem to be lining up these days to tell us that care standards are low and declining, that there are still too many children staying for too long, that new carers are practically impossible to find, that foster children are becoming more and more difficult to manage, and that 'a quagmire of child-swallowing bureaucracies plague the system' (Roche 2000, p. 82). After three years of research into the subject, we too can see much that is critical about foster care. Of particular concern to us is the growing reliance on foster care throughout the western world at a time when the pool of volunteer labour is shrinking under the social and economic forces described in Chapter 3. This clash between demand for and supply of foster carers accounts for much that is wrong with the system. It helps to explain why children are sometimes unhappy or even abused in care, why desperate social workers 'stretch' the truth (see Chapter 12), why overburdened carers leave the system and why so many placements break down. Unless the pressure is relieved, the foster care system in Australia and elsewhere must eventually collapse under the sheer weight of numbers piled on fewer and fewer shoulders. Not only is the absolute number of foster children increasing throughout the western world but data presented in Chapter 3 suggest that the concentration of disruptive children like those described in Chapters 11 and 12 is also on the increase; and we have presented both quantitative and qualitative evidence of the enormous burdens involved in caring for such children.

An increasingly common solution to the state's difficulties in mounting foster care services is to contract out the task to the non-government sector. But at least in the Australian jurisdiction, the problems in foster care have, if anything, been compounded by the extension of the quasi-market to out-of-home care. Although the policy objectives of greater professionalism and accountability within government and non-government agencies are laudable

enough, we have seen for ourselves some of the unintended negative consequences that ensue when agencies which had once been partners in the
service of children suddenly become competing 'suppliers' under highly prescriptive, time-limited service contracts. Among the most troubling of these
consequences has been the demoralizing erosion of inter-sectoral relations
that was reported in Chapters 3 and 5.

Despite the systemic problems besetting foster care today, however, our
results suggest that the service is not 'in crisis' at the level of individual
service recipients. Apart from the obvious benefits to foster children of
security and freedom from harm, the majority of our sample displayed improved psychosocial functioning during their time in care. More specifically,
placement in foster care was found to be associated with declines in the
short term in emotional distress and hyperactivity as well as improvements
in the child's behaviour at home and at school. Furthermore, for those
children who remain in care for the medium to longer term, these short-term
gains also tend to be sustained for the remainder of their time in care. In the
absence of a non-foster-care control group, we cannot know whether these
gains are better or worse than might otherwise be expected, but we can at
least say that there is no evidence of psychological deterioration among
children in long-term foster care. Besides, we have first-hand evidence in
support of foster care. Generally speaking, our consumer feedback studies
showed that foster children report very high levels of satisfaction with the
care they receive and with the social workers who supervise them. We also
found that satisfaction with foster care was significantly correlated with the
carer's score on a standardized measure of care giving behaviour and, surprisingly, scores on this measure were actually higher within our sample of
foster carers than they were for a normative sample of parents from the
general population caring for their own children. Since the care giving instrument was completed by the children in both cases, it is possible that
some or all of the difference can be explained by demand characteristics
operating more on foster children than on natural children, but the fact that
our foster carers performed so well in the eyes of their foster children is a
most encouraging finding none the less. The other significant predictor of
child satisfaction in foster care was the perceived strictness of the carer, with
lower scores on this measure being associated with higher levels of child
satisfaction. This latter result is very reminiscent of research reviewed in
Chapter 1 showing that successful foster parenting is associated with liberal
personality traits, such as: tolerance, a non-authoritarian child-rearing style,
non-possessiveness, rejection of the belief that child development is dependent on heredity and low demand on foster children for religious observance.

Myth 2: Impermanence is harmful to children

Undoubtedly one of the most strident and influential myths in the foster
care field concerns the imperative of placement permanence. As discussed in

Chapter 10, alarm over this issue can be traced back almost half a century to Maas and Engler's (1959) finding that American children placed in what was intended to be temporary foster care often remained there for long periods, neither returning to their families nor settling into a stable alternative. In more recent times, Richard Gelles (in Hughes 1999) spoke for many in the field when he said that the persistence of 'foster care drift' in contemporary America (read also the United Kingdom and Australia) shows that

> child welfare workers look at the world through the eyes of their client – the adult. 'This mother deserves a chance.' Well, what about this kid who's only going to be one year old *once*? What about all the brain cells that have to develop *that year*? That have to be wired *that year*? They don't get a chance to be rewired *next year* – they're wired then. That's a developmental *fact* – a biological neurological *fact*. [emphasis in original]

The philosophy of permanency planning (see Chapters 1 and 10) which is so influential in the United States and the United Kingdom, and which is now gaining ground in Australia as well, represents the formal policy response to the problem of foster care drift. The policy accepts that children will be actively harmed if they are subjected to temporary or unstable living arrangements other than for very short periods of time during which a crisis is either resolved or averted. Under the policy, social workers must begin making plans from the outset of foster placement *both* for the speedy return of children to their families of origin *and* for the termination of parental rights via adoption if the former proves impossible within a reasonable period of time. But this directive begs fundamental questions such as what constitutes a 'reasonable' time frame, and how we balance the need for permanence against potentially competing values such as respecting children's views or finding the optimal placement. In some jurisdictions, the time frame for adoption has even been hard-wired in legislation, but the justification for the period chosen is rarely if ever provided. As Gelles's impassioned statement demonstrates, the public debate (not to mention public policy) in relation to permanency planning tends to be driven more by purple prose than by hard data.

Our own high rate of sample retention after two years shows that foster care in Australia can hardly be considered a temporary way of life for most of the children who enter it. In fact, more of the children in our sample remained within the foster care system than returned home over the period (see Chapter 7). Not only were 46 per cent of our original sample still in foster care two years after the study began, but around half of these had also not managed to find a stable placement after all that time in care (see Chapter 7). Not surprisingly, most placement disruption occurred soon after referral into care but for more than one in five of our sample placement disruption continued for at least two years: 'at least' because around half of the sample had been in care for varying lengths of time before the study began. It is therefore no exaggeration to describe around 20 per cent of our sample as effectively homeless in foster care. Such findings suggest that the state of affairs described by Maas and Engler (1959) in the United States all those years ago applies in Australia today. More importantly for our present purposes the level of placement disruption identified in this study provided us with an ideal opportunity to delineate the social and psychological sequelae of placement instability over varying lengths of time and for different reasons.

Contrary to expectations, our results showed that placement instability for up to at least the eight-month point in care was not in fact associated with psychological harm in the sample as a whole (see Chapter 10). Indeed, repeated placement change over that period was associated with a psychological trajectory that was indistinguishable from children who settled into one foster placement right away. Even more surprisingly, it was only the children who began in unstable placements but then settled down who showed signs of psychosocial deterioration up to the eight-month point (see Chapter 10 for a fuller discussion of these results). Among the inferences that can be drawn from these findings is that the ideal placement is not always achieved on the first attempt and that the only sure way of knowing whether or not a particular arrangement will work is to try it out. It follows that if a placement is unsuccessful or a better opportunity presents itself, foster care workers have nothing to fear from moving the child until, through a process of elimination, the best available option is found. There is, of course, no argument that it is always better to find a stable foster placement from the outset, but it also follows from our findings that this objective should not be elevated to an end in itself. The data therefore sound a timely warning to policy-makers whose anxiety about placement instability is increasingly being translated into sometimes arbitrary performance targets that impose financial penalties for changing placements.

The positive psychosocial outcomes reviewed earlier among children in care for at least two years also questions the common assumption that long-term foster care itself is antithetical to psychological adjustment irrespective of the level of placement stability because it consigns the child to the level of provisional family member. As Lahti's (1982) work (reviewed in Chapter 10) demonstrates, however, the attitudes of the carer and the child's sense of belonging are ultimately what determines the child's sense of family, not the child's legal status. Similarly, the results of our psychological assessments combined with the children's feedback on placement (see Chapter 7) suggest that children can both develop in a positive direction and feel at home in long-term foster care without necessarily terminating parental rights through adoption.

Naturally there are limits on the type and amount of instability that children can tolerate before psychosocial harm is done, and some of our findings help to identify what those limits are. In the first place, we found that, from about the twelve-month point onwards, placement instability is associated with psychosocial deterioration. The second and closely related finding in this regard is that children whose placement disruption was attributable to the behaviour of the child himself or herself were at greatest risk of developmental decline. These findings are related because, if placement instability continues to the twelve-month point, the likelihood of placement change due to disruptive behaviour increases. To put this another way, by the time they go much beyond about eight months in care, most of the children who have moved for positive reasons, such as being closer to family and friends or finding a better school, will have settled down and the proportion of behaviourally disordered children still in unstable placements will therefore have risen. For this reason, the proportion of foster placements that are unstable at or beyond the eight-month point provides an obvious, albeit rough, indicator for foster care providers eager to assess their performance against an empirically derived benchmark. At the level of individual children, we can be even more precise about the type and level of placement disruption that is likely to be acceptable. In short, our results suggest that, after two placement breakdowns due to behaviour, the future course of placement disruption and psychological deterioration becomes so predictable that, as a rule of thumb, children who experience two such breakdowns should normally be removed from conventional family-based foster care and offered something different (see Chapter 11).

The suggestion that disruptive children should be removed from foster care obviously raises the question of what alternatives exist when these same children are among the least likely to return to their biological parents (see Chapter 11) and are also the most unattractive to potential adoptive parents. In addition to residential care, of course, there are numerous other models of out-of-home care that can be tried. Among the best evaluated of them is Therapeutic Foster Care. Therapeutic Foster Care (TFC) appeared in the United States as early as the mid-1970s when it was introduced as an alternative to placing conduct-disordered children and adolescents in institutional care. The definition of TFC remains imprecise. According to Snodgrass (1989), for example, it is simply a family-based programme in which the foster carer is responsible for implementing individualized treatment including 'a stated, measurable goal, a written set of procedures for achieving the goal, and a process for regularly assessing the result' (p. 79). Galaway (1989), on the other hand, considers that the emphasis of TFC is on adjustment to family living rather than on treating the child within a family context.

International surveys of TFC (Bryant 1981; Snodgrass and Bryant 1989) suggest that its treatment interventions tend to be based on numerous therapeutic approaches, but all of them have as a hallmark highly individualized services tailored to fit the needs of programme participants and their families (Clark et al. 1993). This individualized approach to service delivery is sometimes referred to as 'wraparound services', and in a survey of over eight hundred self-designated TFC programmes Hudson, Nutter and Galaway (1990) managed to extract a number of key features common to most of them. Among the most significant of these were:

- The carers are chosen specifically to deal with the most difficult children in care.
- TFC carers receive a higher rate of payment than traditional foster carers and are contracted as employees by the relevant agency.
- TFC carers undergo longer and more intensive training than do regular foster carers.
- TFC carers also receive in-service training.
- Carers normally have only one child at a time placed with them.
- The caseload of the agency support worker is reduced to reflect the extra support required by TFC carers.

The outcome research into TFC varies in methodological rigour (see Hudson, Nutter and Galaway 1994, for a review). Generally speaking, those few adequately controlled trials that have been conducted (e.g. Chamberlain and Reid 1991) have used very small samples. Fanshel, Finch and Grundy's (1990) study of the Casey Family Program included over 580 children but did not employ random allocation. Studies by Hazel (1989), Osmond (1992), and Smith (1986) involved post-test-only measures without control conditions. Another four studies were quasi-experiments with repeated measures (Colton 1988; Fanshel, Finch and Grundy 1990; Hawkins, Almeida and Samet 1989; Thomlison 1991). Methodological shortcomings notwithstanding, the available evidence suggests that the benefits of TFC include reductions in the likelihood of placement breakdown (Fanshel, Finch and Grundy 1990) and offending (Davis et al. 1997) as well as improvements in psychological adjustment (Clark et al. 1993; Colton 1988; Hazel 1989; Osmond 1992). As a result, Meadowcroft, Thomlison and Chamberlain (1994) and Hudson, Nutter and Galaway (1994) have suggested that TFC should be used as an alternative to institutionalization for very difficult children like those described in Chapters 10 and 11.

While Multisystemic Therapy (MST) is actually an alternative to out-of-home care rather than a form of it, it nevertheless deserves mention in the present context because it is a form of intensive therapy that targets the children who are most at risk of 'serial eviction' (see Chapter 11) from foster care. The multisystemic approach views individuals as being surrounded by a network of interconnected systems that encompass individual, family, and extra-familial (peer, school, neighbourhood) factors (Huey et al. 2000). Thus, intervention is often necessary in a combination of these systems, and MST strives to promote behaviour change in the adolescent's natural environment, using the strengths of each system (family, peers, school, neighbourhood, etc.) to facilitate change. MST is provided in the child's own home, which assists family retention and enhances generalization of gains to the natural environment. The usual duration of MST treatment is around sixty hours over four months, but the frequency and duration of sessions are tailored to the needs of children and their families. According to Henggeler *et al.* (1998), one of the best-demonstrated effects of MST is reduction in the need for out-of-home care.

Whole-of-family foster care is another option for disruptive children that has been used in Europe in particular (Barth 2001). In one programme described by Nelson (1992), homeless families referred from local emergency shelters are linked to families who have been specially recruited by state human service workers. All of the foster families have themselves experienced poverty, and their role is to work with the professional human service workers to assist homeless families to meet housing, education, parenting and self-care goals. Though hosted families are responsible for their own basic needs, host families are compensated for their efforts. The programme has four central components. The first is *contracting*, which begins with a family conference. All parties draw up an initial case plan and meet again at three-month intervals to set goals and performance measures for all key stakeholders. The second is *networking*, which attempts to build host parents into the ongoing social networks of the hosted families. The third is a *peer support system* which sees hosted families and their hosts meet in separate settings with their peers. The primary purpose of the meetings is to provide mutual support, but professional facilitators also give presentations on topics such as family communication, housing resources, money management and parenting. Finally, the programme attempts to *mobilize community resources* such as parenting groups and health services. Nelson (1992) claims that the programme has considerable potential in preventing foster placements for disadvantaged children but so far there have been no outcome studies to support this contention. Barth and Price (1999) describe several programmes in the United States which place young mothers and their infants in TFC or with trained resource parents who provide nurturing and skills development. The studies cited have successful programme completion rates ranging from 85 per cent to over 99 per cent, the outcome measure being mother and child remaining together after leaving the programme. Other programmes work with adult parents and their children to reunify the family, to prevent placement, or to enable the parents to consider placing their children for adoption. Outcomes are reported to be better than for families not entering such programmes; however, no details are provided. And in Australia, Jackson (1996) has described a whole-family care programme known as The Family Admission Program in which families are assisted over six months to reunify and/or to avoid foster placement. During the first three months the whole family lives in an independent but intensively supported unit, and the last three months are spent at home with home-based interventions. While in the unit, families have access to support twenty-four hours a day, and family care worker contact ranges from two to eight hours each day. Social workers see the family at least twice a week and support and consult with family care workers on a daily basis. After return home, contact is reduced over time to once or twice a week. If support is still needed at the conclusion of the programme, long-term less intensive services are arranged. Intervention includes work on household and child care routines, discipline, play, supervision and safety, communication, conflict resolution, etc. It is reported that of 17 families referred for reunification, 11 were successful and 10 were still together up to two years later. Once again, lack of comparison with non-treatment families limits the conclusions that can be drawn from his report.

Whatever alternative is considered, however, our findings demonstrate that persisting with foster care for disruptive children (operationally defined as two or more breakdowns due to behaviour) is most unlikely to bring success in the longer term. For everyone else, instability up to about the eight-month point need not necessarily be a contra-indication for foster care.

Myth 3: Parental visiting promotes reunification

In a sense, the myth of parental visiting is a stalking horse for ideological opponents of permanency planning. This is because the staunchest advocates of parental visiting are those who are least likely to approve of terminating parental rights through adoption. In fact, proponents of parental visiting often justify their opposition to the termination of parental rights on the alleged connection between parental contact and child well-being (see below). In Chapter 8, we provided an overview of the research evidence in support of this link between parental visiting and family reunification. We suggested then that much of this work once again boils down to a statistical correlation between the two phenomena. In particular, Fanshel and Shinn's (1978) landmark study found that consistently high rates of parental contact were associated with greatest likelihood of reunification and consistently low rates with least likelihood and that variations up or down over time were associated with increases or decreases in likelihood respectively. The authors also reported that frequency of parental contact seemed to decline the longer children remained in care. Importantly, this aspect of their work was based on the observation that the cohort that remained in care for a short time tended to be visited more often than the cohort that stayed longer. Putting all of these findings together, the foster care field has come to the conclusions that degree of parental contact influences likelihood of reunification and that children need to be protected from long-term foster care wherever possible because their parents stop visiting them after a while. Strictly speaking, of course, Fanshel and Shinn's study did not show that parental contact declines over time but rather that samples that remain in care longer tend to be made up of an increasingly larger proportion of children with little or no contact (see Chapter 8). The only sure way to confirm that parental contact declines over time is to restrict the analysis to children who have been in care for a long period and to examine how often they have been visited throughout their time in care. Confirmation of Fanshel and Shinn's view would come from showing that the children still in care at time 2 had received more frequent contact at time 1 than at time 2.

Some but not all of Fanshel and Shinn's findings were replicated in the present study, and we have questioned the myth attributed to their work that parental visiting increases the likelihood of reunification. Consistent with Fanshel and Shinn (1978), we found a strong and consistent correlation between visiting and reunification, although we did not find that variations in rate of contact altered the likelihood of reunification. Moreover, we found no evidence that parental visiting declines over time. The discrepancies between us on these points could be due at least in part to differences in our sampling frames. Whereas Fanshel and Shinn's (1978) were children new to care, 45 per cent of our sample was made up of children who were already in care and for whom parental contact schedules were already fairly set. More importantly, when we searched explicitly for predictors of reunification, we found that they were mainly what we have referred to as 'external' factors associated with neglect, particularly maternal incapacity due to illness or substance misuse (see Chapter 9). Under these circumstances, it would clearly be naive to focus on frequency of parental visits under the assumption that it will do much to enhance reunification. Bluntly, the data as a whole suggest that more functional families visit more often and more reliably and, not surprisingly, these families are also the most likely to be reunified.

Parental visiting promotes child well-being

Like the reunification myth, the argument that parental visiting promotes child well-being is largely founded on the known statistical correlation between the phenomena (see, for example, Cantos, Gries and Slis, 1996). Among the most sophisticated work of this kind was Fanshell and Shinn's (1978) longitudinal study which found that frequently visited children made greater gains in emotional adjustment than infrequently visited children between intake and two and a half years in care, although this trend did not persist beyond the two-and-a-half-year point. Moreover, the effect of parental visiting on child behaviour was uneven across the different periods. In the present study, frequent parental visiting was associated with measures of psychological well-being, but only in the short term. In the longer term (after two years in care), the association between parental contact and well-being became *negative* for children who had entered care for the first time when the study began, while *change* in frequency of visiting between four months and two years was not associated with change in emotional well-being. These too are correlational findings, and there is no suggestion that parental contact produces psychological improvements in the short term or decrements in the long term. In the long term, for example, it could be that psychological distress causes parents to visit more often and therefore that, if parental visiting were reduced for children in long-term care, their distress could be even greater. All we can confidently say is that among those children who remain in care for long periods, frequent parental contact is associated with lower levels of psychological adjustment. Further research is clearly needed to uncover the explanation for this phenomenon and to identify any causal connections operating between the relevant variables. What is clear, however, is that it would be unwise to adopt a blanket policy of promoting parental contact under the assumption that this will promote child well-being and compensate for family separation.

Conclusion

This chapter has been titled 'Myths and Legends in Foster Care' not 'Fallacies in Foster Care' because, like all myths, those we have reviewed do contain some half-truths. There is indeed a growing crisis in foster care, but this is related more to social and demographic trends than it is to inherent deficiencies in foster care, as a form of out-of-home care. It is also true that a certain kind and length of placement impermanence is antithetical to child development, but not all forms of 'instability' are harmful. Moreover, while parental visiting is associated both with reunification and, in the short term, with child well-being as well, data presented in this book also call for important qualifications to the parental visiting myths identified. Like all myths, those reviewed above tend to be highly simplified ways of viewing things and they can have disastrous consequences when uncritically applied to the real world. The solution, of course, is not to jettison the mythology altogether because most of it is partly accurate in some circumstances. Rather, the foster care field needs to move to a more sophisticated set of practice principles which take account of situational and individual difference variables such as those identified in the pages of this book.

References

Achenbach, T. M. (1991) *Manual for the Child Behavior Checklist 4–18 and 1991 Profile*. Burlington, VT: University of Vermont, Department of Psychology.

Aday, L. A. and Anderson, R. (1975) *Access to Medical Care*. Ann Arbor: Health Administration Press.

Adcock, M. (1980) The right to a permanent placement. *Adoption and Fostering*, 99, 21–4.

Ainsworth, F. (1997) Foster care research in the US and Australia. An update. *Children Australia*, 22, 9–16.

Aldgate, J. and Hawley, D. (1986) Helping foster families through disruption. *Adoption and Fostering*, 10, 44–9.

Altshuler, S. J. and Gleeson, J. P. (1999) Completing the evaluation triangle for the next century: measuring child 'wellbeing' in family foster care. *Child Welfare*, 78, 125–47.

American Humane Association (1993) *First National Roundtable on Outcome Measures in Child Welfare Services*. Englewood, CO: Author.

Andersson, G. (1999) Children in permanent foster care in Sweden. *Child and Family Social Work*, 4, 174–86.

Association of Children's Welfare Agencies (1991) Standards in foster care. Retrieved 10 August 2001 from http://www.acwa.asn.au/

Australian Broadcasting Corporation (1999) Crisis in care for state wards as foster parents overwhelmed, 15 October. http://www.abc.net.au/7.30/stories/s59766.htm

Australian Bureau of Statistics (1999) *Australian Social Trends*. Canberra: Australian Government Publishing Service.

Australian Bureau of Statistics (2002) *2002 Labour Statistics*. Canberra: Author. Catalogue No. 6104.0.

Australian Institute of Health and Welfare (2000) *Child Protection Australia 1998–99*. AIHW cat. no. CSW 11. Canberra: AIHW (Child Welfare Series no. 25)

Barber, J. G. (2003) *Social Work Through the Lifecycle*. Melbourne: Tertiary Press.

—— (in press) Australian industrial relations policy and workers with family responsibilities. *Community, Work and Family*.

Barber, J. G., Bolitho, F. and Bertrand, I. (1999a) The predictors of adolescent smoking. *Journal of Social Services Research*, 26, 51–66.

—— (1999b) Intrapersonal versus peer group predictors of adolescent drug use. *Children and Youth Services Review*, 21, 565–79.

Barber, J. G. and Delfabbro, P. H. (2000a) The standardized assessment of child well-being in child protection work. *The Journal of Social Work Research and Evaluation*, 1, 111–23.

—— (2000b) Predictors of adolescent adjustment: parent–peer relationships and parent–child conflict. *Child and Adolescent Social Work Journal*, 17, 275–88.

Barber, J. G., Delfabbro, P. H. and Cooper, L. L. (2000) Aboriginal and non-Aboriginal children in out-of-home care. *Children Australia*, 25, 5–10.

—— (2001) The predictors of unsuccessful transition to foster care. *The Journal of Child Psychology and Psychiatry*, 42, 785–90.

Barth, R. P. (1997) Foster family care. In J. D. Berrick, R. Barth and N. Gilbert (eds), *Child Welfare Research Review*, vol. 2. New York: Columbia University Press.

—— (2001) Policy implications of foster family characteristics. *Family Relations: Interdisciplinary Journal of Applied Family Studies*, 50, 16–19.

Barth, R. P. and Berry, M. (1987) Outcomes of child welfare services under permanency planning. *Social Service Review*, 61, 71–90.

Barth, R. P. and Price, A. (1999) Shared family care: providing services to parents and children placed together in out-of-home care. *Child Welfare*, 78, 88–197.

Barth, R. P., Yeaton, J. and Winterfelt, N. (1994) Psychoeducational groups with foster parents of sexually abused children. *Child and Adolescent Social Work Journal*, 11, 405–24.

Baum, A. C., Crase, S. J. and Crase, K. L. (2001) Influences on the decision to become or not become a foster parent. *Families in Society*, 82, 202–13.

Bebbington, A. and Miles, J. (1990) The supply of foster families for children in care. *British Journal of Social Work*, 20, 283–307.

Bell, M. (1998) The Looking After Children materials. *Adoption and Fostering*, 22, 15–23.

Benedict, M. I. and White, R. B. (1991) Factors associated with foster care length of stay. *Child Welfare*, 70, 45–58.

Benedict, M. I., White, R. B., Stallings, R. and Cornely, D. A. (1989). Racial differences in health care utilization among children in foster care. *Children and Youth Services Review*, 11, 285–97.

Benedict, M. I., Zuravin, S., Brandt, D. and Abbey, H. (1994) Types and frequency of child maltreatment by foster care providors in an urban population. *Child Abuse and Neglect*, 18, 577–85.

Benedict, M. I., Zuravin, S. and Stallings, R. (1996) Adult functioning of children who lived in kin versus nonrelative family foster homes. *Child Welfare*, 75, 529–49.

Berkley-Hill, B. (1988) *The Challenge of Foster Care*. London: National Foster Care Association.

Berrick, J. D. (1997) Assessing quality of care in kinship and foster family care. *Family Relations*, 46, 273–80.

Berrick, J. D. and Barth, R. P. (1994) Research on kinship foster care: what do we know? Where do we go from here? *Children and Youth Services Review*, 16, 1–6.

Berrick, J. D., Barth, R. P. and Needle, B. (1994) A comparison of kinship foster homes and foster family homes: implications for kinship foster care as family preservation. *Children and Youth Services Review*, 16, 33–64.

Berridge, D. and Cleaver, H. (1987) *Foster Home Breakdown*. Oxford: Basil Blackwell.

Berry, M. (1988) A review of parent training programs in child welfare. *Social Service Review*, 62 (2), 302–23.

—— (1992) An evaluation of family preservation services: fitting agency services to family needs. *Social Work*, 37, 314–21.

Bilson, A. and Barker, R. (1995) Parental contact with children fostered and in residential care after the Children Act 1989. *British Journal of Social Work*, 25, 367–81.

Blome, W. (1997) What happens to foster kids: educational experiences of a random sample of foster care youth and a match group of non-foster care youth. *Child and Adolescent Social Work Journal*, 14, 41–53.

Bowlby, J. (1969) *Attachment*. London: Hogarth Press.

Boyd, L. H. and Remy, L. L. (1978) Is foster-parent training worthwhile? *Social Service Review*, 52 (2), 275–96.

Boyd, P. E. (1979) They can go home again. *Child Welfare*, 58, 605–15.

Boyle, M. and Jones, S. (1985) Selecting measures of emotional and behavioral disorders of children for use in general populations. *Journal of Child Psychology and Psychiatry*, 26, 137–59.

Boyle, M. H., Offord, D. T., Hofman, H. G., Catlin, G. P., Byles, J. A., Cadman, D. T., Crawford, J. W., Links, P. S., Rae-Grant, N. I. and Szatmari, P. (1987) Ontario Child Health Study: I. Methodology. *Archives of General Psychiatry*, 44, 826–31.

British Broadcasting Corporation News (1999) Social services ordered to improve, 20 September. http://news.bbc.co.uk/1/hi/uk/572946.stm

—— (2000) Care children still at risk of abuse, 10 January. http://news.bbc.co.uk/1/hi/uk/wales/596810.stm

Bryant, B. (1981) Special foster care: a history and rationale. *Journal of Clinical Child Psychology*, 1, 8–20.

Bryce, M. E. and Ehlert, R. C. (1971) 144 foster children. *Child Welfare*, 50, 499–503.

Buchanan, A. (1995) Young people's views on being looked after in out-of-home care under the Children Act 1989. *Children and Youth Services Review*, 17, 681–96.

Bullock, R., Little, M. and Millham, S. (1993) *Going Home: The Return of Children Separated from their Families*. Aldershot: Dartmouth.

Burdekin, B. (1989) *Our Homeless Children: Report of the National Inquiry into Homeless Children*. Canberra: Australian Government Publishing Service.

Burry, C. L. (1999) Evaluation of a training program for foster parents of infants with prenatal substance effects. *Child Welfare*, 78, 197–214.

Butler, S. and Charles, M. (1999) 'The past, the present, but never the future': thematic representations of fostering disruption. *Child and Family Social Work*, 4, 9–19.

Campbell, C. and Downs, S. W. (1987) The impact of economic incentives on foster parents. *Social Service Review*, 599–609.

Cantos, A. L., Gries, L. T. and Slis, V. (1996) Behavioral correlates of parental visiting during family foster care. *Child Welfare*, 76 (2), 309–29.

Carbino, R. (1980) *Foster Parenting: An Updated Review of the Literature*. New York: Child Welfare League of America.

Casey Family Program (2000) Lighting the way: attracting and supporting foster families. www.casey.org/cnc/documents/lighting the way full doc.pdf

Cautley, P. W. and Aldridge, M. J. (1975) Predicting success for new foster parents. *Social Work*, 20, 48–53.

Chamberlain, P., Moreland, S. and Reid, K. (1992) Enhanced services and stipends for foster parents: effects on retention rates and outcomes for children. *Child Welfare*, 71, 387–401.

Chamberlain, P. and Reid, J. (1991) Using a specialized foster care community treatment model for children and adolescents leaving the state mental hospital. *Journal of Community Psychology*, 19, 266–76.

—— (1994) Differences in risk factors and adjustment for male and female delinquents in treatment foster care. *Journal of Child and Family Studies*, 3, 23–39.

Charlesworth, S. (1996) *Stretching Flexibility: Enterprise Bargaining, Women Workers and Changes to Working Hours*. Sydney: Human Rights and Equal Opportunity.

Child Welfare League of America (1988) *Standards for Health Care Services for Children in Out-of-Home Care*. Washington, DC: Author.

—— (1991) *A Blueprint for Fostering Infants, Children, and Youths in the 1990s*. Washington, DC: Author

Claburn, W. E., Magura, S. and Resnick, W. (1976) Administrative case review for foster care: a brief national assessment. *Child Welfare*, 55, 395–405.

Clare, M. (1997) The UK 'Looking After Children' project: fit for 'out-of-home care' practice in Australia? *Children Australia*, 22, 29–35.

Clark, H., Boyd, L., Redditt, C., Foster-Johnson, L., Hardy, D., Kuhns, J. *et al.* (1993) An individualized system of care for foster children with behavioral and emotional disturbances: preliminary findings. In K. Kutash, C. Liberton, A. Algarin and R. Friedman (eds), *Fifth Annual Research Conference Proceedings for a System of Care for Children's Mental Health* (pp. 365–70). Tampa, FL: University of Southern Florida.

Clark, H. B., Prange, M. E., Lee, B., Boyd, L. A., McDonald, B. A. and Stewart, E. S. (1994) Improving adjustment outcomes for foster children with emotional and behavioral disorders: early findings from a controlled study on individualized services. *Journal of Emotional and Behavioral Disorders*, 2, 207–18.

Cleaver, H. (1997) Contact: the social workers' experience. *Adoption and Fostering*, 21, 34–40.

Cliffe, D. and Berridge, D. (1991) *Closing Children's Homes: An End to Residential Child Care*. London: National Children's Bureau.

Cohen, J. (1992) A power primer. *Psychological Bulletin*, 112, 155–9.

Colton, M. (1988) *Dimensions of Substitute Child Care*. Aldershot: Avebury.

Colton, M. and Williams, M. (1997) The nature of foster care: international trends. *Adoption and Fostering*, 21, 44–9.

Combs-Orme, R., Chernoff, R. G. and Kager, V. A. (1991) Utilization of health care by foster children: application of a theoretical model. *Children and Youth Services Review*, 13, 113–29.

Community Services Commission (2000) *Voices of Children and Young People in Foster Care: Report from a Consultation with Children and Young People in Foster Care in New South Wales*. Sydney: Author.

Courtney, M. E. (1993) Standardized outcome evaluation of child welfare services out-of-home care: problems and possibilities. *Children and Youth Services Review*, 15, 349–69.

—— (1994) Factors associated with the reunification of foster children with their families. *Social Service Review*, 68, 81–108.

—— (1995a) Reentry to foster care of children returned to their families. *Social Service Review*, 69, 226–41.

—— (1995b) The foster care crisis and welfare reform. *Public Welfare*, Summer, 27–33.

—— (1996) Kinship foster care and children's welfare: the California experience. *Focus*, 17, 42–7.

Courtney, M. E. and Barth, R. (1996) Pathways of older adolescents out of foster care: implications for independent living services. *Social Work*, 41, 75–83.

Courtney, M. E. and Wong, Y. I. (1996) Comparing the timing of exits from substitute care. *Children and Youth Services Review*, 18, 307–34.

Coyne, A. and Brown, M. (1986) Relationship between foster care and adoption units serving developmentally disabled children. *Child Welfare*, 64, 189–98.

Cross, J. (1990) Substitute Care for Children with Disabilities. Adelaide: Unpublished report.

Cunningham, M. and Freeman, R. (1993) Young people leaving care: the challenge. In *Proceedings of 23rd AASW National Conference*, ed. J. Gaha. Australian Association of Social Workers, Canberra, 72–7.

Curtis, P. A., Dale, G. and Kendall, J. C. (eds) (1999) *The Foster Care Crisis*. Lincoln and London: University of Nebraska Press in association with the Child Welfare League of America.

Dando, I. and Minty, B. (1987) What makes good foster parents? *British Journal of Social Work*, 17, 383–400.

Davidson, B. (1997) Service needs of relative caregivers: a qualitative analysis. *Families in Society*, 78, 502–10.

Davis, J. W., Pecora, P. J., Joyce, C., Flemmer, L., Edmondson, J., Gerhardt, J., *et al.* (1997) The design and implementation of family foster care services for high risk delinquents. *Juvenile and Family Court Journal*, 48, 17–42.

De Groot, M. E. (1981) *Backgrounds of Children in Residential Care and the Development of Placements: Follow-up Onderzoek*. Deventer, Netherlands: Jeugd Onder Dak.

Denby, R., Rindfleisch, N. and Bean, G. (1999) Predictors of foster parents' satisfaction and intent to continue to foster. *Child Abuse and Neglect*, 23, 287–303.

Denley, L. and Wilson, L. (1993) *Project to Address the Issues Concerning Children with Disability Unable to Continue to Live in the Family Home*. Adelaide: Family and Community Services.

Department of Family and Community Services (1995) *Annual Report, 1994–95*. Adelaide: Author.

—— (1996) *A Policy for the Planning, Purchasing and Delivery of Alternative Care Services in South Australia*. Adelaide: Author.

—— (1997) *Fostering*. Adelaide: Author.

Department of Health (2002) Fostering for the future: inspection of foster care services. Available at http://www.doh.gov.uk/ssi/fosteringaw.pdf

Dickey, B. (1980) *No Charity There: A Short History of Social Welfare in Australia*. Melbourne: Thomas Nelson Australia.

Dini, J. and Olivieri, R. (1993) *A Discussion of Review Findings about Foster Care Services in South Australia: The Macro View*. Adelaide: Family and Community Services.

Doelling, J. L. and Johnson, J. H. (1990) Predicting success in foster placement: the contribution of parent–child temperament characteristics. *American Journal of Orthopsychiatry*, 60, 585–93.

Drury-Hudson, J. (1995) Maintaining links: resource demands and social work attitudes in respect to parent–child access in a statutory child welfare agency. *Children Australia*, 20, 18–23.

Dubowitz, H. (1994) Kinship care: suggestions for future research. *Child Welfare*, 73, 553–64.

Dubowitz, H., Feigelman, S., Harrington, D., Starr, R., Zuravin, S. and Sawyer, R. (1994) Children in kinship care: how do they fare? *Children and Youth Services Review*, 16, 85–106.

Dubowitz, H., Feigelman, S. and Zuravin, S. (1993) A profile of kinship care. *Child Welfare*, 69, 513–22.

English, D. J., Kouidou-Giles, S. and Plocke, M. (1994) Readiness for independence: a study of youth in foster care. *Children and Youth Services Review*, 16, 147–58.

Everett, J. E. (1995) Relative foster care: an emerging trend in foster care policy placement and practice. *Smith College Studies in Social Work*, 65, 239–54.

Fahlberg, V. (1992) *A Child's Journey through Placement*. London: BAAF.

Family and Community Services (1995) *Annual Report, 1994–95*. Adelaide: Author.

—— (1997) *Practice Guidelines*. Adelaide: Author.

Family and Youth Services (1999) Family and Youth Services Manual. Available at www.sacentral.sa.gov.au/agencies/fays.

Fanshel, D. (1975) Parental visiting of foster children in foster care: key to discharge? *Social Service Review*, 49, 493–514.

—— (1979) Preschoolers entering foster care in New York City: the need to stress plans for permanency. *Child Welfare*, 58 (2), 67–87.

Fanshel, D., Finch, S. J. and Grundy, J. F. (1989) Modes of exit from foster family care and adjustment at time of departure of children with unstable life histories. *Child Welfare*, 68, 391–402.

—— (1990) *Foster Children in a Life Course Perspective*. New York: Columbia University Press.

Fanshel, D. and Shinn, E. (1978) *Children in Foster Care: A Longitudinal Investigation*. New York: Columbia University Press.

Farmer, E. (1992) Restoring children on court orders to their families: lessons for practice. *Adoption and Fostering*, 16, 7–15.

—— (1993) Going home – what makes reunification work? In P. Marsh and J. Triseliotis (eds), *Prevention and Reunification in Child Care*. London: Batsford.

—— (1996) Family reunification with high risk children: lessons from research. *Children and Youth Services Review*, 18, 403–18.

Farmer, E. and Parker, R. (1991) *Trials and Tribulations: Returning Children from Local Authority Care to their Families*. London: HMSO.

Fein, E. and Maluccio, A. (1984) Children leaving foster care: outcomes of permanency planning. *Child Abuse and Neglect*, 8, 425–31.

Fein, E., Maluccio, A. N., Hamilton, V. J. and Ward, D. E. (1983) After foster care: outcomes of permanency planning for children. *Child Welfare*, 62, 485–562.

Fein, E., Maluccio, A. N. and Kluger, M. (1990) *No More Partings: An Examination of Long-term Foster Family Care*. Washington, DC: Child Welfare League of America.

Ferguson, T. (1966) *Children in Care and After*. Oxford: Oxford University Press.

Fernandez, E. (1999) Pathways in substitute care: representation of placement careers of children using event history analysis. *Children and Youth Services Review*, 21, 177–216.

Festinger, T. (1983) *Nobody Ever Asked Us . . . a Postscript to Foster Care*. New York: Columbia University Press.

—— (1994) *Returning to Care: Discharge and Reentry in Foster Care*. Washington, DC: Child Welfare League of America.

Fisher, T., Gibbs, I., Sinclair, I. and Wilson, K. (2000) Sharing the care: the qualities sought of social workers by foster carers. *Child and Family Social Work*, 5, 225–33.

Forward, A. and Carver, M. (1999) The reunification of South Australian children with their families: case characteristics and outcomes. Paper presented at the seventh Australasian Conference on Child Abuse and Neglect, Perth, Western Australia.

Fratter, J., Rowe, J., Sapsford, D. and Thoburn, J. (1991) *Permanent Family Placement: A Decade of Experience*. London: BAAF.

Frost, R. (1915) *North of Boston*. New York: Henry Holt and Company.

Fuller-Thomson, E. and Minkler, M. (2000) The mental and physical health of grandmothers who are raising their grandchildren. *Journal of Mental Health and Aging*, 6, 311–23.

Galaway, B. (1989) Toward a definition of specialist foster care. *Community Alternatives: International Journal of Family Care*, 1, 82–4.

Gambrill, E. D. and Wiltse, K. T. (1974) Foster care: prescriptions for change. *Public Welfare*, 39–47.

Garrett, P. M. (1999) Mapping child-care social work in the final years of the twentieth century: a critical response to the 'Looking After Children' system. *British Journal of Social Work*, 29, 27–47.

Gean, M. P., Gillmore, J. L. and Dowler, J. K. (1985) Infants and toddlers in supervised custody: a pilot study of visitation. *Journal of the American Academy of Child Psychiatry*, 24, 608–12.

Gendell, S. J. (2001) In search of permanency: a reflection on the first 3 years of the Adoption and Safe Families Act. *Family Court Review*, 39, 25–42.

General Accounting Office (1995) *Foster Care: Health Needs of Many Young Children are Unknown and Unmet*. GAO/HEHS-95-114. Washington, DC: US Government Printing Office.

Gibbs, S. (1996) Community care – the next 20 years (Workforce Issues). *Proceedings of Community Care: The Next 20 Years. A Future Policy Conference*. Canberra: Carers Association of Australia.

Gibson, T. L., Tracy, G. S. and DeBord, M. S. (1984) An analysis of the variables affecting length of stay in foster care. *Children and Youth Services Review*, 6, 135–45.

Gilbertson, R. and Barber, J. G. (2002) Obstacles in involving children and young people in foster care research. *Child and Family Social Work*, 7 (4), 253–8.

—— (in press) Placement breakdown among disrupted adolescents: cover perspectives and system factors. *Australian Social Work*.

Gillespie, J. M., Byrne, B. and Workman, L. J. (1995) An intensive reunification program for children in foster care. *Child and Adolescent Social Work Journal*, 12, 213–28.

Gilligan, R. (1996) The foster carer experience in Ireland: findings from a postal survey. *Child: Care, Health and Development*, 22, 82–98.

—— (2000) The importance of listening to the child in foster care. In G. Kelly and R. Gilligan (eds), *Issues in Foster Care*. London: Jessica Kingsley Publishers.

Glezer, H. (1991) Juggling work and family commitments. *Family Matters*, 28, 6–11.

Glisson, C. (1994) The effect of services coordination teams on outcomes for children in state custody. *Administration in Social Work*, 18, 1–23.

Goerge, R. M. (1990) The reunification process in substitute care. *Social Service Review*, 64, 422–57.

Govan, E. (1951) A community program of foster home care in N.S.W. *Social Service Review*, 25, 363–75.

Green, R. G., Braley, D. and Kisor, A. (1996) Matching adolescents with foster mothers and fathers: an evaluation of the role of temperament. *Journal of Child and Family Studies*, 5, 267–83.

Grigsby, R. K. (1994) Maintaining attachment relationships among children in foster care. *Families in Society*, 75, 269–76.

Hahn, A. (1994) The use of assessment procedures in foster care to evaluate readiness for independent living. *Children and Youth Services Review*, 16, 171–9.

Hair, J. F., Anderson, R. E., Tatham, R. L. and Black, W. C. (1995) *Multivariate Data Analysis* (4th edn). Englewood Cliffs, NJ: Prentice Hall.

Hawkins, R., Almeida, C. and Samet, M. (1989) Comparative evaluation of foster-family-based family treatment and five other placement choices: a preliminary report. In A. Algarin, R. Friedman, A. Duchnowski, K. Kutah, S. Silver and M. Johnson (eds), *Children's Mental Health Services and Policy: Building a Research Base* (pp. 98–119). Proceedings of the Second Annual Research Conference, Research and Training Center for Children's Mental Health, University of South Florida, Florida Mental Health Institute, Tampa, FL.

Hayden, C., Goddard, J., Gorin, S. and van der Spek, N. (1999) *State Child Care: Looking after Children?* London: Jessica Kingsley Publishers.

Hazel, N. (1989) Adolescent fostering as a community resource. *Community Alternatives: International Journal of Family Care*, 1, 47–52.

Heath, A. F., Colton, M. J. and Aldgate, J. (1994) Failure to escape: a longitudinal study of foster children's educational attainment. *British Journal of Social Work*, 24, 241–60.

Hegar, R. L. (1988) Sibling relationships and separations: implications for child placement. *Social Service Review*, 62, 446–66.

Henggeler, S. W., Mihalic, S. F., Rone, L., Thomas, C. and Timmons-Mitchell, J. (1998) *Blueprints for Violence Prevention, Book Six: Multisystemic Therapy*. Boulder, CO: Center for the Study and Prevention of Violence.

Henry, D., Cossett, D., Auletta, T. and Egan, E. (1991) Needed services for foster parents of sexually abused children. *Child and Adolescent Social Work*, 8, 127–40.

Hess, P. (1982) Parent–child attachment concept: crucial for permanency planning. *Social Casework*, 63, 46–53.

—— (1988) Case and context: determinants of planned visit frequency in foster family care. *Child Welfare*, 67, 311–25.

Hess, P. M., Folaron, G. and Jefferson, A. B. (1992) Effectiveness of family reunification services: an innovative evaluative model. *Social Work*, 37, 305–11.

Hess, P., Mintun, G., Moelhman, A. and Pitts, G. (1992) The Family Connection Center: an innovative visiting program. *Child Welfare*, 71, 77–88.

Hess, P. and Proch, K. (1988) Contacts between birth families and foster children. *Journal of Child Psychology and Psychiatry*, 38, 581–6.

Hicks, C. and Nixon, S. (1989) The use of a modified repertory grid technique for assessing the self-concept of children in local authority foster care. *British Journal of Social Work*, 19, 203–16.

Hilmer, F., Rayner, M. and Tapperell, G. (1993) *National Competition Policy: Report of the Independent Committee of Inquiry into Competition Policy in Australia (Hilmer Report)*. Canberra: Australian Government Publishing Service.

Hochstadt, N. J., Jaudes, P. A., Zimo, D. A. and Schachter, J. (1987) The medical and psychological needs of children entering foster care. *Child Abuse and Neglect*, 11, 53–62.

Holman, R. (1973) The place of fostering in social work. *British Journal of Social Work*, 5, 3–29.

Hornby, H. C. and Collins, M. I. (1981) Teenagers in foster care: the forgotten majority. *Children and Youth Services Review*, 3, 7–20.

Hudson, J., Nutter, R. and Galaway, B. (1990) Specialist foster family-based care: North American developments. In B. Galaway, D. Maglajklic, J. Hudson, P. Harmon and J. McLagan (eds), *International Perspectives on Specialist Foster Family Care*. St Paul, MN: Human Service Associates.

—— (1992) A survey of North American specialist foster family care programs. *Social Service Review*, 66, 50–63.

—— (1994) Treatment foster care programs: a review of evaluation research and suggested directions. *Social Work Research*, 18, 198–210.

Huey, S. J., Henggeler, S. W., Brondino, M. J. and Pickrel, S. G. (2000) Mechanisms of change in multisystemic therapy: reducing delinquent behavior through therapist adherence and improved family and peer functioning. *Journal of Counsulting and Clinical Psychology*, 68 (3), 451–67.

Hughes, S. (1999) The children's crusaders. *The Pennsylvania Gazette*, May/June, 22–9.

Inglehart, A. (1993) Adolescents in foster care: predicting behavioral maladjustment. *Child and Adolescent Social Work Journal*, 6, 521–32.

—— (1994) Adolescents in foster care: predicting readiness for independent living. *Children and Youth Services Review*, 16, 159–69.

Industry Commission (1997) *Reforms in Government Service Provision. Case Studies: Human Services in South Australia, Public Hospitals in Victoria, Correctional Services in Queensland*. Melbourne: Author.

Jackson, A. (1996) The Reconnections and Family Admission Programs: two models for family reunification within Melbourne, Australia. *Community Alternatives*, 8, 53–75.

Jenkins, S. and Diamond, B. (1985) Ethnicity and foster care: census data as predictors of placement variables. *American Journal of Orthopsychiatry*, 55, 267–76.

Jenkins, S. and Norman, E. (1969) Families of children in foster care. *Children*, 16, 155–9.

Jennings, M. A., McDonald, T. and Henderson, R. A. (1996) Early citizen review: does it make a difference? *Social Work*, 41, 224–31.

Jivanjee, P. (1999) Professional and provider perspectives on family involvement in Therapeutic Foster Care. *Journal of Child and Family Studies*, 8, 329–41.

Johnson, P. R., Yoken, C. and Voss, R. (1995) Family foster care placement: the child's perspective. *Child Welfare*, 74, 959–74.

Jones, E. (1975) A study of those who cease to foster. *British Journal of Social Work*, 5, 31–41.

Jones, J., Clark, R., Kufeldt, K. and Norman, M. (1998) *Looking After Children*: assessing outcomes in child care. The experience of implementation. *Children and Society*, 12, 212–22.

Jones, M. and Jones, B. (1983) *West Virginia's Former Foster Children: Their Experiences in Care and Their Lives as Young Adults*. New York: Child Welfare League of America.

Katz, L. (1990) Effective permanency planning for children in foster care. *Social Work*, 35, 220–6.

Keogh, L. and Svensson, U. (1999) Why don't they become foster carers? A study of people who inquire about foster care. *Children Australia*, 24 (2), 13–19.

Kilmartin, C. (1997) Home-based work: snapshots from recent labour market trends. *Family Matters*, 47 (winter), 20–3.

Kinard, E. M. (1994) Methodological issues and practical problems in conducting research on maltreated children. *Child Abuse and Neglect*, 18, 645–56.

Klee, L. and Halfon, N. (1987) Mental health care for foster children in California. *Child Abuse and Neglect*, 11, 63–74.

Klee, L., Soman, L. A. and Halfon, N. (1992) Implementing critical health services for children in foster care. *Child Welfare*, 71, 99–111.

Knight, T. and Caveney, S. (1998) Assessment and action records: will they promote good parenting? *British Journal of Social Work*, 28, 29–43.

Kosonen, M. (1996) Maintaining sibling relationships – neglected dimension in child care practice. *British Journal of Social Work*, 26, 809–22.

Kufeldt, K. (1984) Listening to children – who cares? *British Journal of Social Work*, 14, 257–64.

Kufeldt, K., Armstrong, J. and Dorosh, M. (1996) Connection and continuity in foster care. *Adoption and Fostering*, 20, 14–20.

Kusserow, R. P. (1992) *Using Relatives for Foster Care*. Department of Health and Human Services. Washington, DC: Office of the Inspector General.

Lahti, J. (1982) A follow-up study of foster children in permanent placements. *Social Service Review*, 56 (4), 556–71.

Lawder, E., Poulin, J. E. and Andrews, R. (1986) A study of 185 foster children five years after placement. *Child Welfare*, 65, 241–5.

Lawrence, R. (1994) Recruiting carers for children in substitute care: the challenge of program revision. *Australian Social Work*, 47, 37–42.

Leashore, B. R. (1986) Workers' perceptions of foster care review in the District of Columbia. *Child Welfare*, 65, 26–32.

Lee, T. (1987) Needs based planning and services for older people. In C. Foster and H. Kendig (eds), *Who Pays: Financing Services for Older People*. Canberra: Commonwealth Policy Coordination Unit and ANU Ageing and Family Project, ANU.

Leifer, M., Shapiro, J. P. and Kassem, L. (1993) The impact of maternal history and behavior upon foster placement and adjustment in sexually abused girls. *Child Abuse and Neglect*, 17, 755–66.

Le Prohn, N. S. (1994) The role of the kinship foster parent: a comparison of the role conceptions of relative and non-relative foster parents. *Children and Youth Services Review*, 16, 65–84.

Le Prohn, N. S. and Pecora, P. J. (1994) The Casey Foster Parent Study research summary. Retrieved 13 August, 2001, from www.casey.org/research/reports/reportsdocs.htm

Lewis, R. E., Walton, E. and Fraser, M. W. (1995) Examining family reunification services: a process analysis of a successful experiment. *Research on Social Work Practice*, 5, 259–82.

Lindsey, E. W. (2001) Foster family characteristics and emotional problems of foster children: practice implications for child welfare, family life education, and marriage and family therapy. *Family Relations*, 50, 19–22.

Link, M. K. (1996) Permanency outcomes in kinship care: a study of children placed in kinship care in Erie County, New York. *Child Welfare*, 75, 509–28.

Littner, N. (1956) *Traumatic Effects of Separation and Placement*. New York: Columbia University Press.

Lowe, M. I. (1991) The challenge of partnership: a National Foster Care Charter. *Child Welfare*, 70, 151–6.

Maas, H. S. and Engler, R. E. (1959) *Children in Need of Parents*. New York: Columbia University Press.

Macaskill, C. (1991) *Adopting or Fostering a Sexually Abused Child*. London: Batsford.

McDonald, T. P., Allen, R. I., Westerfelt, A. and Piliavin, I. (1996) *Assessing the Long-term Effects of Foster Care*. Washington, DC: Child Welfare League of America Press.

McLean, J. (1999) Foster care crisis needs attention. *The Topeka Capital-Journal*, 17 February.

McMillen, J. C., Rideont, G. B., Fisher, R. H. and Tucker, J. (1997) Independent living services: the views of former foster youth. *Families in Society*, 78, 471–88.

Magura, S. and Moses, B. S. (1986) *Outcome Measures for Child Welfare Services: Theory and Applications*. Washington, DC: Child Welfare League of America.

Mallon, G. (1992) Junior life skills: an innovation for latency-age children in out-of-home care. *Child Welfare*, 71, 585–91.

Mallon, G. P. (1998) After care, then where? Outcomes of an independent living program. *Child Welfare*, 77, 61–78.

Maloney, T. (1994) Has New Zealand's Employment Contracts Act increased employment and reduced wages? *Economic Working Paper, No. 135*. University of Auckland.

Maluccio, A. N. and Fein, E. (1985) Growing up in foster care. *Children and Youth Services Review*, 7, 123–34.

Maluccio, A. N., Fein, E. and Davis, P. (1994) Family reunification: research findings, issues and directions. *Child Welfare*, 73, 489–504.

Maluccio, A. N., Fein, E. and Olmstead, K. A. (1986) *Permanency Planning for Children: Concepts and Methods*. New York: Tavistock Publications.

Maluccio, A. N., Warsh, R. and Pine, B. A. (1993) Rethinking reunification after foster care. *Community Alternatives: International Journal of Family Care*, 5, 1–17.

Maunders, D., Liddell, M. and Green, S. (1999) *Young People Leaving Care and Protection: A Report to the National Youth Affairs Research Scheme*. Hobart: Australian Clearinghouse for Youth Studies.

Meadowcroft, P. and Grealish, E. M. (1990) Training and supporting treatment parents. In P. Meadowcroft and B. A. Trout (eds), *Troubled Youth in Treatment Homes: A Handbook of Therapeutic Foster Care*. Washington, DC: Child Welfare League of America.

Meadowcroft, P., Thomlison, B. and Chamberlain, P. (1994) Treatment foster care services: a research agenda for child welfare. *Child Welfare*, 73, 565–81.

Mech, E. V. (1985) Parental visiting and foster placement. *Child Welfare*, 64, 67–72.

Mech, E. V., Ludy-Dobson, C. and Hulseman, F. S. (1994) Life-skills knowledge: a survey of foster adolescents in three placement settings. *Children and Youth Services Review*, 16, 181–200.

Mech, E. V. and Rycroft, J. R. (eds) (1995) *Preparing Foster Youths for Independent Living: Proceedings of an Invitational Research Conference*. Washington, DC: Child Welfare League of America.

Meier, E. G. (1966) Adults who were foster children. *Children*, 13, 16–22.

Mellor, D. and Storer, S. (1988) Support groups for children in alternate care: a largely untapped therapeutic resource. *Child Welfare*, 74, 905–18.

Mendes, P. and Goddard, C. (2000) Leaving care programs locally and internationally: towards better outcomes. *Children Australia*, 25, 11–16.

Miedema, B. and Nason-Clark, N. (1997) Foster care redesign: the dilemma contemporary foster families face. *Community Alternatives*, 9, 15–28.

Miller, P. M., Gorski, P. A., Borchers, D. A., Jenista, G. A. *et al.* (2000) Developmental issues for young children in foster care. *Pediatrics*, 106, 1145–50.

Millham, S., Bullock, R., Hosie, K. and Haak, M. (1986) *Lost in Care: The Problem of Maintaining Links Between Children in Care and their Families*. Aldershot: Gower.

Milner, J. L. (1987) An ecological perspective on duration of foster care. *Child Welfare*, 66, 113–23.

Minnis, H., Pelosi, A. J., Knapp, M. and Dunn, J. (2001) Mental health and foster carer training. *Archives of Disease in Childhood*, 84, 302–6.

Minty, B. (1999) Annotation: outcomes in long-term foster family care. *Journal of Child Psychology and Psychiatry*, 40, 991–9.

Nelson, K. M. (1992) Fostering homeless children and their parents too: the emergence of whole family foster care. *Child Welfare*, 71, 575–84.

Nelson, R. H., Singer, M. J. and Johnsen, L. O. (1978) The application of a residential treatment evaluation model. *Child Care Quarterly*, 7, 164–73.

New South Wales Department of Community Services (1998) New South Wales Standards for Substitute Care Services. Retrieved on 10 August 2001 from http://www.community.nsw.gov.au/progpub.htm

Nixon, S. (1997) The limits of support in foster care. *British Journal of Social Work*, 27, 913–30.

Nugent, W. R., Carpenter, D. and Parks, J. (1993) A statewide evaluation of family preservation and family reunification services. *Research on Social Work Practice*, 3 (1), 40–65.

Orme, J. G. and Buehler, C. (2001) Foster family characteristics and behavioral and emotional problems of foster children: a narrative review. *Family Relations*, 50, 3–15.

Osborn, A. (2002) Foster carer's perceptions of the effects of parental contact upon the psychosocial wellbeing of the child. Unpublished Honours thesis, Department of Psychology, University of Adelaide, South Australia.

Osmond, M. (1992) *The Treatment Foster Care Program for the Children's Aid Societies of Durham, Kawartha-Haliburton, and Northumberland*. Coburg, ON: Ontario Association of Children's Aid Societies and the Ministry of Community and Social Services.

Palmer, S. E. (1990) Group treatment of foster children to reduce separation conflicts. *Child Welfare*, 69, 227–38.

—— (1996) Placement stability and inclusive practice in foster care: an empirical study. *Children and Youth Services Review*, 18, 589–601.

Pardeck, J. T. (1983) An empirical analysis of behavioral and emotional problems of foster children as related to re-placement in care. *Child Abuse and Neglect*, 7, 75–8.

—— (1984) Multiple placement of children in foster family care: an empirical analysis. *Social Work*, Nov.–Dec., 506–9.

Parker, R., Ward, H., Jackson, S., Aldgate, J. and Wedge, P. (eds) (1991) *Looking After Children: Assessing Outcomes in Child Care*. London: HMSO.

Pecora, P., Fraser, M. W., Haapala, D. and Barlome, I. A. (1987) *Defining Family Preservation Services: Three Intensive Home-based Treatment Programs*. Salt Lake City: University of Utah, Social Research Institute.

Pithouse, A. and Parry, O. (1997) Fostering in Wales. *Adoption and Fostering*, 21, 41–9.

Poulin, J. (1985) Long term foster care, natural family attachment and loyalty conflict. *Journal of Social Service Research*, 9, 17–29.

—— (1992) Kin visiting and the biological attachment of long-term foster children. *Journal of Social Service Research*, 15, 65–79.

Proch, K. and Howard, J. A. (1986) Parental visiting of children in foster care. *Social Work*, May–June, 178–81.

Quiggin, J. (1998) Social democracy and market reform in Australia and New Zealand. *Oxford Review of Economic Policy*, 14:1 (spring), 76–98.

Rapp, C. A. and Poertner, J. (1987) Moving clients center stage through the use of client outcomes. *Administration in Social Work*, 11, 23–38.

Ray, J. and Horner, W. C. (1990) Correlates of effective therapeutic foster parenting. *Residential Treatment for Children and Youth*, 7, 57–69.

Reed, J. (1997) Fostering children and young people with learning disabilities. *Adoption and Fostering*, 20, 36–41.

Reeuwijk, P. M. and Berben, E. G (1988) *Voluntary Foster Care. A Quantitative Analysis*. The Hague, Netherlands: CWOK.

Reid, W. J., Kagan, R. M. and Schlosberg, S. B. (1988) Prevention of placement: critical factors in program success. *Child Welfare*, 67, 25–36.

Rest, E. R. and Watson, K. W. (1984) Growing up in foster care. *Child Welfare*, 63, 291–306.

Rhodes, K. W., Orme, J. G. and Buehler, C. (2001) A comparison of family foster parents who quit, consider quitting, and plan to continue fostering. Retrieved on 20 April 2002 from: http://web1.infotrac.galegroup.com/itw

Robbins, J. (1997) Playing a symphony or playing a market? A South Australian perspective on contracting for care. *Third Sector Review*, 3, 67–97.

Robinson, M. M., Kropf, N. P. and Myers, L. (2000) Grandparents raising grandchildren in rural communities. *Journal of Mental Health and Aging*, 6, 353–65.

Roche, T. (2000) The crisis of foster care. *Time Magazine*, 13 November.

Rowe, D. C. (1976) Attitudes, social class, and the quality of foster care. *Social Service Review*, 50, 506–14.

Rowe, J., Hundleby, M. and Garnett, L. (1989) *Child Care Now*. London: British Agencies for Adoption and Fostering.

Ryan, P., McFadden, E. J., Rice, D. and Warren, B. (1988) The role of foster parents in helping young people develop emancipation skills. *Child Welfare*, 67, 563–72.

Rzepnecki, T. L. (1987) Recidivism of foster children returned to their own homes: a review and new directions for research. *Social Services Review*, 61, 56–70.

Sanchirico, A. L., Lau, W. J., Jablonka, K. and Russell, S. J. (1998) Foster parent involvement in service planning: does it increase job satisfaction? *Children and Youth Services Review*, 20, 325–46.

Sandow, M. E. (1998) Subsystem variables associated with positive foster mother–foster child relationships [Abstract]. *Dissertation Abstracts International Section B The Sciences and Engineering*, 58, 5655.

Scannapieco, M., Hegar, R. L. and McAlpine, C. (1997) Kinship care and foster care: a comparison of characteristics and outcomes. *Families in Society*, 78, 480–7.

Scannapieco, M., Schagrin, J. and Scannapieco, T. (1995) Independent living programs: do they make a difference? *Child and Adolescent Social Work Journal*, 12, 381–9.

Schofield, G., Beek, M. and Sargent, K. (2000) *Growing up in Foster Care*. London: BAAF.

Scholte, E. M. (1997) Exploration of criteria for residential and foster care. *Journal of Child Psychology, Psychiatry and Allied Health*, 38, 657–66.

Schuerman, L. R., Rzepnecki, T. L. and Johnson, P. R. (1994) *Outcomes in Evaluation of the Family First Reunification Program of the Department of Children and Family Services, Final Report*. Chicago: Chaplin Hall Centre for Children, University of Chicago.

Schwab, A., Bruce, M. and Mercy, R. (1986) Using computer technology in child placement decisions. *Social Casework*, 67, 359–68.

Seaberg, J. R. and Tolley, E. S. (1986) Predictors of length of stay in foster care. *Social Work Research and Abstracts*, 22, 11–17.

Segal, U. A. and Schwartz, S. (1985) Factors affecting placement decisions of children following short-term emergency care. *Child Abuse and Neglect*, 9, 543–8.

Shadbolt, N. and Burton, M. (1990) Knowledge elicitation. Chapter 13 in J. R. Wilson and E. N. Corlett (eds), *Evaluation of Human Work*. London: Taylor & Francis.

Shapiro, D. (1976) *Agencies and Foster Children*. New York: Columbia University Press.

Simms, M. D. and Bolden, B. J. (1991) The family reunification project: facilitating regular contact among foster children, biological families, and foster families. *Child Welfare*, 70, 679–90.

Smith, B. (1988) Something you do for love: the question of money and foster care. *Adoption and Fostering*, 12, 34–9.

Smith, E. P. and Gutheil, R. H. (1998) Successful foster parent recruiting: a voluntary agency effort. *Child Welfare*, 67, 137–46.

Smith, M. C. (1994) Child rearing practices associated with better developmental outcomes in preschool-age foster children. *Child Study Journal*, 24, 299–326.

Smith, P. (1986) Evaluation of Kent placements. *Adoption and Fostering*, 10, 22–33.

Snodgrass, R. (1989) Treatment foster care: a proposed definition. *Community Alternatives: International Journal of Family Care*, 1, 79–82.

Snodgrass, R. and Bryant, B. (1989) Therapeutic foster care: a national program survey. In R. Hawkins and J. Breiling (eds), *Therapeutic Foster Care: Critical Issues*. Washington, DC: Child Welfare League of America.

Staff, I. and Fein, E. (1992) Together or separate: a study of siblings in foster care. *Child Welfare*, 71, 257–70.

Steinhauer, P. D., Johnston, M., Hornick, J. P., Barker, P., Snowden, M. *et al.* (1989) The Foster Care Research Project: clinical impressions. *American Journal of Orthopsychiatry*, 59, 430–41.

Stone, J. (1991) The tangled web of short-term foster care: unravelling the strands. *Adoption and Fostering*, 15, 4–9.

Stone, M. (1989) *Young People Leaving Care: A Study of Management Systems Service Delivery and User Evaluation*. Royal Philanthropic Society.

Stone, N. M. and Stone, S. F. (1983) The prediction of successful foster placement. *Social Casework*, 64, 11–17.

Stuntzner-Gibson, D., Koren, P. E. and DeChillo, N. (1995) The youth satisfaction questionnaire: what kids think of services. *Families in Society*, 76 (10), 614–24.

Substitute Care Reference Group (1994) *Out-of-Home Care in South Australia*. Adelaide: Department of Family and Community Services.

Taber, M. and Proch, K. (1987) Placement stability for adolescents in foster care: findings from a program experiment. *Child Welfare*, 66, 433–45.

Tam, T. S. K. and Ho, M. K. W. (1996) Factors influencing the prospect of children returning to their parents from out-of-home care. *Child Welfare*, 75, 253–68.

Taylor, D. and Starr, P. (1967) Foster parenting: an integrative review of the literature. *Child Welfare*, 46, 371–85.

Taylor, J. (1990) *Leaving Care and Homelessness*. Melbourne: Brotherhood of St Laurence.

Teather, E. C., Davidson, S. D. and Pecora, P. (1999) Placement disruption in family foster care. Retrieved on 2 February 2002 from: http://www.casey.org/research/pdisrupt/html

Teishroeb, R. (1999) Foster care system becomes grim game of musical chairs. *Seattle Post-Intelligence Reporter*, 23 September.

Thomas, N. and O'Kane, C. (1999) Children's participation in reviews and planning meetings when they are 'looked after' in middle childhood. *Child and Family Social Work*, 4, 221–30.

Thomlison, B. (1991) Family continuity and stability of care: critical elements in treatment foster care programs. *Community Alternatives*, 3, 1–18.

Thorpe, M. B. and Swart, G. T. (1992) Risk and protective factors affecting children in foster care: a pilot study of the role of siblings. *Canadian Journal of Psychiatry*, 37, 616–22.

Thorpe, R. (1974) 'Mum and Mrs. So and So'. *Social Work Today*, 4, 22.

Titterington, L. (1990) Foster care training: a comprehensive approach. *Child Welfare*, 69, 157–65.

Triseliotis, J. (1980) Growing up in foster care and after. In J. Triseliotis (ed.), *New Developments in Foster Care and Adoption*. London: Routledge & Kegan Paul.

Triseliotis, J. and Russell, J. (1984) *Hard to Place: The Outcome of Adoption and Residential Care*. London: Heinemann.

Turner, J. (1984) Reuniting children in foster care with their biological parents. *Social Work*, 29, 501–5.

US Department of Health and Human Services (2000) Adoption and foster care analysis and reporting system (AFCARS). www.acf.ahhs.gov/programs/cb/stats/tarreport/rpt0100/ar0100.htm

Usher, C. L., Randolph, K. A. and Gogan, H. C. (1999) Placement patterns in foster care. *Social Service Review*, 73, 22–36.

Van der Oever, A. C., Hoogheid, B. J. and Hirschfeldt, L. J. (1979) *Placement in Foster Care*. Leiden, Netherlands: University of Leiden.

Weinstein, E. (1960) The self image of the foster child. New York: Russell Sage Foundation.

Wells, K. and D'Angelo, L. (1994) Specialized foster care: voices from the field. *Social Service Review*, March, 127–44.

Wert, E. S., Fein, E. and Haller, W. (1986) 'Children in Placement' (CIP): a model for citizen-judicial review. *Child Welfare*, 65, 199–201.

Whittaker, J. K., Tripodi, T. and Grasso, A. J. (1990) Youth and family characteristics: treatment histories, and service outcomes: some preliminary findings from the Boysville research program. *Child and Youth Services Review*, 16, 139–53.

Wilson, L. and Conroy, J. (1999) Satisfaction of children in out-of-home care. *Child Welfare*, 78, 53–69.

Wise, S. (1999) *The UK Looking After Children Approach in Australia*. Melbourne: Australian Institute of Family Studies.

Wit, O. C. and Adriani, P. J. A. (eds) (1971) *Research in Foster Care*. Utrecht, Netherlands: University of Utrecht.

Wulczyn, F. H. and Goerge, R. M. (1992) Foster care in New York and Illinois: the challenge of rapid change. *Social Service Review*, June, 278–94.

Yeabsley, J. and Savage, J. (1996) The New Zealand labour market: comment on recent developments. *Proceedings of the 25th Annual Conference of Economists*. Canberra: Australian National University.

Zill, N. and Coiro, M. J. (1992) Assessing the condition of children. *Children and Youth Services Review*, 14, 119–36.

Zimmerman, R. (1982) Foster care in retrospect. *Tulane Studies in Social Welfare*, 14, 1–119.

Index